Nutrition and Dietetics for Nurses

Mary E. Beck

Formerly Senior Therapeutic Dietitian,
The Royal Belfast Hospital for Sick Children;
Therapeutic Dietitian, Royal Victoria Hospital, Belfast
and St Bartholomew's Hospital, London;
Teacher of Domestic Science in England and Northern Ireland

Revised by

Helen M. Barker BSc SRD

Research Dietitian,
Department of Gastroenterology and Nutrition,
Central Middlesex Hospital, London

With a contribution by

Helen A. Attrill SRN

Nurse Nutritionist,
Department of Gastroenterology and Nutrition,
Central Middlesex Hospital, London

SEVENTH EDITION

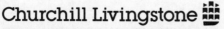
Churchill Livingstone
EDINBURGH LONDON MELBOURNE AND NEW YORK 1985

CHURCHILL LIVINGSTONE
Medical Division of Longman Group UK Limited

Distributed in the United States of America by Churchill Livingstone Inc., 1560 Broadway, New York, N.Y. 10036, and by associated companies, branches and representatives throughout the world.

First edition 1962
Second edition 1965
Third edition 1971
Fourth edition 1975
Fifth edition 1977
Sixth edition 1980
Seventh edition 1985
 Reprinted 1986

ISBN 0-443-03121-5

British Library Cataloguing in Publication Data
Beck, Mary E.
  Nutrition and dietetics for nurses. — 7th ed.
  — (Churchill Livingstone nursing texts)
  1. Diet therapy
  I. Title   II. Barker, Helen M.
  III. Attrill, Helen A.
  615.8'54'024613   RM216

Library of Congress Cataloging in Publication Data
Beck, Mary E.
  Nutrition and dietetics for nurses.
  (Churchill Livingstone nursing texts)
  Includes index.
  1. Diet therapy. 2. Nutrition. 3. Nursing.
I. Barker, Helen M. II. Attrill, Helen A. III. Title.
IV. Series.   [DNLM: 1. Dietetics — Nurses' instruction.
2. Nutrition — Nurses' instruction. WB 400 B393n]
RM216.B364 1985 613.2'024613   84–5873

Produced by Longman Group (FE) Ltd
Printed in Hong Kong

9-35

Nutrition and Dietetics for Nurses

613.2 | BEC

nourished

CHURCHILL LIVINGSTONE NURSING TEXTS

Preface to the First Edition

To the nurse the science of nutrition should prove an interesting and rewarding subject of study as its practical application is to her a matter of day-to-day experience. In her work she has many opportunities of influencing people and helping them towards better eating habits. In illness the patient becomes dependent upon those who are caring for him and is often amenable to suggestions to which formerly he would have paid no attention. Because she has the confidence of her patients the nurse may be able to bring about a permanent improvement in their eating habits.

The provision of a well-balanced hospital dietary sets a good example and establishes an association between good nutrition and restoration to health. Here again the influence of the nurse can be effective, as she represents the needs of the patients to the catering establishment.

Modifications of the diet are employed in the treatment of many diseases and in some cases may be the only form of treatment available. It is not easy to carry out these modifications successfully unless the nurse has a sound knowledge of the principles involved.

The nurse exerts a considerable influence in her community, and a knowledge of the principles of nutrition and how to apply them will prove to be one of her most effective weapons in the fight against disease.

Belfast, 1962   M.E.B.

Postcript
Since publication of the sixth edition I have retired, but I have been very happy to hand over responsibility for updating this edition to Mrs Barker and Miss Attrill. I hope the new team will have the same success and satisfaction that involvement with the book gave me.

Preface to the Seventh Edition

In recent years there has been a growing public awareness of both the importance of good nutrition for health and the role of nutrition in the prevention and treatment of disease. New objective evidence is accumulating rapidly which puts nutrition on a much more scientific basis than ever before. It is essential that all those involved in health care should have a sound knowledge and clear understanding of the principles of nutrition and of their application in dietetics. Nurses, in particular, have close contact with patients, which provides many opportunities to educate them towards better eating habits.

In revising this book I have incorporated much new information on general nutrition and on nutrition and disease. Some aspects are controversial, but on these I have tried to give a balanced view. All the chapters have been thoroughly revised and updated in the light of recent advances. In addition, each chapter begins with a summary and concludes with questions.

There are seven new chapters dealing with areas of growing importance in nutrition in the 1980s. Dietary fibre is of sufficient importance to be considered separately in Chapter 8. Diseases caused by, or associated with, particular diets are discussed in Chapter 9. Dietary recommendations for adults are often taken for granted. These have been clarified in

Chapter 13. Nutritional problems in the elderly and in ethnic minorities are increasing and are considered in Chapters 14 and 15. The importance of diet in dental disease is discussed separately in Chapter 17. Chapter 21 includes a new section on enteral and parenteral nutrition which has been written by a nurse nutritionist. It discusses the practical problems of intensive nutritional therapy which are now being encountered in most branches of nursing.

This revision and updating which incorporates many new developments in nutrition and dietetics will, I trust, enhance the value of this book for nurses and other health care workers.

I would like to thank Dr Rodney H. Taylor of the Department of Gastroenterology and Nutrition for his help and encouragement in the preparation of this edition.

London, 1985

H.M.B.

Contents

1

Introduction to nutrition

Before proceeding to the study of nutrition it is necessary to introduce and explain various terms which are used in connection with the subject.

Nutrition may be described as the sum of the processes by which a living organism receives materials from its environment and uses them to provide its own vital activities. Such materials are known as nutrients.

Nutrients. This term is commonly applied to any substance which is digested and absorbed and used to promote body function. These nutrients may be classified as protein, fat, carbohydrate, minerals, vitamins and water.

Essential nutrient. This is a nutrient which is necessary for life and cannot be synthesised by the body, therefore it must be included in the diet.

Diet. This is the selection of foods which are normally eaten by a person or population.

Food. This is a substance that when eaten, digested and absorbed, provides at least one nutrient.

Balanced diet. This is a diet which provides adequate amounts of all nutrients—not too much and not too little.

Malnutrition occurs when the diet contains an incorrect amount of one or more nutrients.

1

Nutritional status is the state of health produced by the balance between requirement and intake of nutrients.

Nutritional assessment: The measurement of nutritional status. This is based on anthropometric and biochemical data and a dietary history.

Dietitian. This is a person who applies the science of nutrition to the feeding of individuals and groups, both in health and disease.

Metabolism

This term is used to describe all the changes which are constantly taking place in the body as a result of tissue activity. The word itself means change, and in the course of metabolism these nutrients take part in many transformations as a result of which energy is liberated, tissue is formed, and the body functions necessary for the maintenance of life are stimulated and controlled. There are two types of metabolism.

1. *Anabolism*: complex molecules are synthesised from simpler ones—this reaction requires energy.
2. *Catabolism*: complex molecules are broken down to simpler ones and energy is released.

The type of metabolism that occurs in growth is anabolism. Catabolism occurs during starvation and illness when the energy intake is inadequate.

A brief outline of the function of nutrients in the body

A rigid classification of the functions of nutrients is impossible because their functions often overlap.

Carbohydrate is broken down by the body to produce heat and energy.

Protein provides material for tissue formation and repair. It can also be broken down to produce energy.

Fats are used to provide heat and energy, some are incorporated into body tissue.

Water provides the fluid medium that is essential for all metabolic processes. It is also necessary for the excretion of waste products and has an important role in temperature regulation.

Minerals and vitamins are important in the regulation of body processes. Minerals are incorporated into some body tissues.

Measurement of nutrients in foods

The majority of foods have been analysed and details of their composition are available. Some common foods are listed in Appendix 4 along with their content of certain important nutrients.

It will be seen that the energy value of foods can be expressed as either calories or joules. The calorie is the more familiar term. It is a unit of heat. The unit used in nutrition is the kilocalorie, often referred to as a calorie for the sake of convenience.

The calorie, however, is not recognised in the International System of Units agreed in 1960. It has been replaced by the joule. The joule is a unit of energy, irrespective of the form in which that energy is manifested; for example it can denote heat, muscular energy, or electrical energy. In nutrition large amounts of energy are being considered, and the most convenient units are the kilojoule and the megajoule, the prefix 'mega' denoting one million.

In the international system of units, substances can be measured in moles (symbol:mol). A mole is the atomic weight, or molecular weight as applicable, of the substance, expressed in grams. For example the molecular weight of sodium chloride is 58.5; 58.5 grams of sodium chloride are therefore 1 mole.

Further information on units of measurement will be found in Appendix 1. The calorie and the joule are discussed in more detail in Chapter 7.

2

Carbohydrates

50 - 55 %

SUMMARY

Carbohydrate provides the major energy source for man. Dietary carbohydrates are starch, sucrose, lactose and fructose. The most important of these is the glucose polysaccharide starch, which is digested by pancreatic amylase.

The final products of carbohydrate digestion are the monosaccharides; glucose, fructose and galactose. Glucose is the most important of these. Glucose metabolism is under hormonal control. Glucose is used to produce energy and excess glucose is converted to glycogen and fat and stored.

An inadequate carbohydrate intake leads to ketosis.

Carbohydrates are compounds consisting of carbon, hydrogen and oxygen. They include starch, and sugar in its various forms. Plants have the ability to produce sugar and starch from the carbon dioxide of the air and water from the soil. Man obtains carbohydrate by the inclusion of plant foods in his diet.

4

Function

Carbohydrate is oxidised in the body to give heat and energy for all forms of body activity. Carbon dioxide and water are formed as end-products and are excreted principally by the lungs and kidneys. One gram of carbohydrate provides 16 kj (4 kcal) on oxidation in the body.

Structure of the carbohydrates

The simplest forms of carbohydrate with which we are concerned in human nutrition are the simple sugars, glucose, fructose and galactose. These are known as monosaccharides. Structure of glucose molecule:

Pairs of monosaccharides combine to form disaccharides. The disaccharides which are most important in human nutrition are sucrose, lactose and maltose. Their composition is illustrated below.

Glucose + fructose –> sucrose
Glucose + galactose –> lactose
Glucose + glucose –> maltose

Structure of sucrose molecule:

Glucose   Fructose

Large numbers of monosaccharides joined together give polysaccharides. The most important polysaccharide in human nutrition is starch, which is composed of many glucose units.

There are two types of starch: amylose and amylopectin.

Amylose consists of a straight chain of 70–350 glucose molecules. Part of an amylose chain is illustrated below.

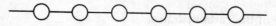

O = 1 glucose molecule

Amylopectin is a branched chain of up to 100 000 glucose molecules.

Sources of carbohydrate

Glucose is prepared commercially from starch and is found in some fruits, notably grapes.

Fructose is found in honey and in fruits; it is sometimes called 'fruit sugar'.

Sucrose is the table sugar we are all familiar with. It is obtained from sugar beet and sugar cane and occurs in some fruits and vegetables.

Lactose is the sugar found in milk.

Galactose does not occur naturally but is produced by the digestion of lactose.

Maltose is found in sprouting grain and is formed during the manufacture of beer.

Starch is the storage carbohydrate produced by plants. Considerable amounts are found in all grains, unripe fruit and certain vegetables such as potatoes, peas, beans and lentils.

Glycogen. Animals store carbohydrate as glycogen in the liver and muscles. Meat is not a dietary source of carbohydrate because the glycogen is destroyed during the hanging process.

Cellulose is a component of plant cell walls. It is found in cereals, vegetables and fruit and is commonly known as fibre. It is not available to the human body as food as there are no digestive secretions present with which to break it down. It is nevertheless a valuable constituent of the diet as it adds bulk to the intestinal contents, stimulating peristalsis and aiding excretion of the faeces.

In the case of herbivorous animals cellulose is available as a food, owing to the presence in the gut of bacteria which convert it to substances which can be absorbed and utilised.

Properties of sugars

An important characteristic of sugars is their sweetness. The degree of sweetness varies with different sugars. They are listed in descending order of sweetness below, fructose being the most sweet and lactose the least sweet.

fructose
sucrose
glucose
maltose
galactose
lactose

All sugars are soluble in water, lactose being the least soluble.

Uses of sugars

Sucrose is used for the most domestic purposes: it is used both as a sweetener and a preservative. Sucrose is added to many manufactured foods to improve the taste, texture and appearance.

Glucose is frequently employed where a high energy intake is required, as it is easily obtained, readily soluble and not so sweet as sucrose, so that larger amounts may be added to foods without imparting an over-sweet flavour.

Fructose is sometimes used as a sweetener by diabetics.

Glucose syrup is made by hydrolysing starch and is used in the food industry, particularly in the manufacture of jams.

Digestion

Starch is broken down to maltotriose, alpha limit dextrins and maltose, principally as a result of the action of pancreatic amylase. The disaccharides are converted to their constituent monosaccharides by the action of disaccharide-splitting enzymes in the small bowel, at the surface of the mucosal cells. These disaccharidases are sucrase, maltase and lactase. Thus available dietary carbohydrates are absorbed into the body in the form of the single sugars, or monosaccharides. Disaccharides are digested rapidly, and sugars are absorbed into the blood stream shortly after being taken by mouth. They therefore provide a more immediate source of energy than starch, which has a longer digestive process to undergo. Different carbohydrate-containing foods are digested and absorbed at different rates. The rate of digestion is influenced by the food form, fibre content and type of carbohydrate.

Absorption and utilisation

After absorption into the capillaries of the intestinal villi the materials resulting from the digestion of carbohydrate (glucose, fructose and galactose) travel to the liver in the portal vein.

These sugars derived from dietary carbohydrate are utilised in three ways.

1. *Metabolised to produce energy.* Much of the glucose leaves the liver in the blood stream and is conveyed around the body to be used as a fuel for the production of energy for cell activity.

2. *Converted to glycogen.* Glycogen is synthesised from glucose in the muscles and stored to be released when it is required for the performance of muscular work. Glycogen is also synthesised by and stored in the liver. Liver glycogen is synthesised from glucose, galactose, fructose and the breakdown products of protein and fat.

3. *Converted to fat.* When muscles and liver are stocked with glycogen, excess carbohydrate is converted to fat, which is stored in the adipose tissues.

Blood sugar level

A certain concentration of glucose is available at all times in the blood, varying between 4.5 and 10 millimoles per litre. This blood sugar level is maintained by the liver, the glycogen stores of which are broken down into glucose and liberated into the blood stream in this form when the level falls below approximately 4.5 millimoles per litre.

In normal circumstances, the blood sugar never rises above approximately 10 mmol per l. In abnormal circumstances, however, and notably in the case of diabetic people who cannot metabolise carbohydrate correctly, the glucose level rises above this figure, in which case the kidneys will excrete the excess. The renal (or kidney) threshold for glucose is said to be 10 mmol per l.

In a small proportion of people the renal threshold is lower than normal and glucose appears in the urine when the level in the blood is not abnormally high. It is important to distinguish this benign condition from diabetes mellitus.

Hormonal control

Certain hormones play a part in the metabolism of carbohydrate. Insulin, secreted by the β cells of the pancreatic islets, is thought to act by assisting the passage of glucose through the cell membrane into the interior, where it is then available for metabolic activity. Adrenaline, secreted by the adrenal medulla, stimulates the release of glucose from the breakdown of glycogen in the liver. Glucagon, from the α cells of the pancreatic islets, also promotes release of glucose from liver glycogen. Growth hormone, from the pituitary gland, antagonises insulin and brings about a rise in blood sugar level.

Daily intake

In United Kingdom diets, carbohydrate accounts for between 40 and 50 per cent of the total energy intake. Figure 2.1 shows the types and sources of carbohydrate in the United Kingdom diet.

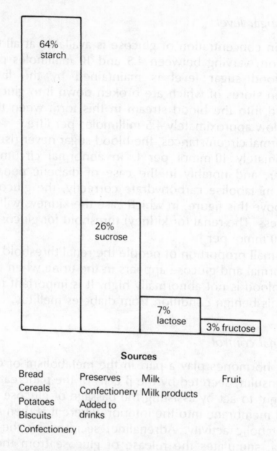

Sources

Bread	Preserves	Milk	Fruit
Cereals	Confectionery	Milk products	
Potatoes	Added to		
Biscuits	drinks		
Confectionery			

Figure 2.1 Sources of carbohydrate in the United Kingdom diet.

Foods high in carbohydrate are plentiful, cheap, palatable, and easily prepared for the table. In the planning of diets it is necessary to ensure in the first place an adequacy of foods of value primarily for their content of proteins, minerals and vitamins. At the same time it should be appreciated that many foods high in carbohydrate, for example potatoes, and bread and other baked products, make an important contribution to the intake of these other nutrients. Reference should be made to Table 4.1.

Unfortunately a substantial part of our carbohydrate is taken in the form of sucrose—sugar as it is found in the sugar bowl and in cakes and confectionery is almost entirely pure carbohydrate.

Excess carbohydrate

1. An excessive intake of carbohydrate usually implies a high sugar intake, and when it exceeds the energy requirements of the body, leads to conversion of the excess carbohydrate to fat, which is stored, giving rise to obesity.

2. It is a common dietary fault in our society to take too much of our carbohydrate in refined form. The indigestible fibre which is present in whole grain cereal foods such as porridge and wholemeal bread is necessary for normal functioning of the bowel. Diets high in sugar and in refined cereal foods such as white bread are correspondingly low in fibre. There is evidence to suggest that such diets contribute to the development of bowel disorders in later life.

3. Diets which are high in carbohydrate, especially sugar, are likely to be lacking in foods containing important amounts of other essential nutrients.

Insufficient carbohydrate

1. Lack of carbohydrate in the diet results in insufficient glucose being available for production of energy, with the result that fat is used to an extent greater then normal. During fat metabolism substances known as ketones are produced. In the absence of sufficient carbohydrate these are produced at a rate exceeding that of their disposal, their accumulation in the body giving rise to a toxic state known as ketosis.

2. The primary function of protein is to build body tissue. However, if a lack of carbohydrate and fat occurs, protein will be diverted from this purpose and used instead to give energy. Carbohydrate is therefore said to be a protein sparer, and lack of carbohydrate can thus cause depletion of body tissue, as in starvation resulting from famine, or from the inability to take food during illness. For maximum protein-sparing action carbohydrate and protein should be taken together at the same meal.

A lack of carbohydrate in the diet is unusual. Under conditions in which the energy requirement is increased, however, as in febrile states and over-activity of the thyroid gland, the usual intake may be insufficient to meet the unusual demand and a state of relative carbohydrate lack occurs.

In diabetes mellitus also the inability of the body cells to utilise glucose produces a lack of carbohydrate at cell level.

QUESTIONS

1. List six carbohydrate rich foods.
2. How does the body digest carbohydrate?
3. What is carbohydrate used for in man?

3

Fats ~~30 - 35 %~~

SUMMARY

Fats provide a concentrated energy source. Fats and oils consist of a combination of glycerol and fatty acids. Most Western diets contain too much fat for good health. Meat and dairy products contain saturated fatty acids; some plant seeds contain polyunsaturated fatty acids. Saturated fats raise serum cholesterol more than polysaturated fats. Fats are emulsified by bile and digested by pancreatic lipase. The products of digestion are metabolised to provide energy, stored in the adipose tissue or incorporated into some of the body tissues.

The structure of fats

Fats, like carbohydrates, are composed of atoms of carbon, hydrogen and oxygen, but arranged in different patterns and proportions. They are formed by the combination of glycerol with fatty acids, each unit of glycerol combining with three fatty acid units to give a triglyceride. Many different fatty acids occur. A triglyceride can contain three identical fatty acids or a mixture of different fatty acids. It is the particular types and combination of fatty acids which give each type of fat its own identity and physical properties. The fats with which we are

13

familiar, for example in butter, dripping and olive oil. are mixtures of triglycerides. Examples of the fatty acids occurring in dietary fats are stearic, palmitic and oleic acids.

1 molecule glycerol + 3 molecules fatty acid →
1 molecule triglyceride (fat) and water

Hydrogenation

The carbon atoms in the hydrocarbon chain of the fatty acid part of the triglyceride molecule can be linked by 'single' or 'double' bonds. If all the bonds are single the fat is called saturated; if double bonds are present the fat is unsaturated. The fatty acids of saturated fats are more stable than those of unsaturated fats. The double bonds in unsaturated fats can be converted to single bonds; this process is known as hydrogenation. This process alters both the chemical structure and the physical properties of the fat, making it harder and raising its melting point. Margarine is produced by the hydrogenation of oils such as palm oil, corn oil and soya oil.

Saturated fats

All bonds in the fatty acid moiety are single, e.g., palmitic and stearic acid, which are found in lard and suet.

Monosaturated fats

These contain one double bond, e.g., oleic acid, which is found in many fats particularly olive oil.

Polyunsaturated fats

These contain more than one double bond, e.g., linoleic acid, which is found in vegetable seed oils such as soya and corn oils.

Hydrogenation: saturated and unsaturated fats

The fatty acids present in most soft fats and oils contain less hydrogen than those in the harder fats and on this account are referred to as being unsaturated. More hydrogen can be introduced into their structure by chemical means. This process is called hydrogenation and results in the formation of a fat firmer in consistency. Margarine, which so much resembles butter in appearance, is prepared by the hydrogenation of oils such as palm oil. Cooking fat, other than lard, is prepared from hydrogenated oils.

Rancidity

Rancidity in fats is due to the liberation of free fatty acids, some of which have a disagreeable odour and flavour, and also to exposure to the oxygen of the air. Unsaturated fats become oxidised more readily than the saturated fats and are therefore more liable to develop rancidity.

Solubility

Fats are insoluble in water but in certain circumstances will form a suspension of minute particles known as an emulsion. This process takes place during the digestion of fats in the intestine.

Sources

Fats are derived from both animal and vegetable sources. Fats which are liquid below 20°C are called oils. Fish and vegetable fats are referred to as oils, as they are liquid at room temperature.

Animal fats include beef dripping, suet, mutton fat and lard (pork fat). They also include the fats of dairy produce—eggs, and milk and its products, cream, butter and cheese. These contain cholesterol, either in the free form or combined with glycerol to form an ester. The tissues of dark-fleshed fish such as herrings, sardines and salmon are oil-containing. Certain fish livers are rich in oil, hence cod liver oil and halibut liver oil.

Vegetable fats include olive oil, coconut oil, palm oil, cotton-seed oil, corn oil and others. These contain plant sterols, which are poorly absorbed, and not cholesterol.

Digestion and absorption

Fat disgestion starts in the duodenum where fats are emulsified by bile and hydrolysed to free fatty acids and monoglycerides by the pancreatic enzyme lipase. The greater proportion of these products of digestion enter the mucosal cells where they reform as triglycerides. Some combine with protein and cholesterol to form lipoproteins. The remainder are absorbed directly into the portal circulation as fatty acids and glycerol.

Functions

1. Source of energy. Fats are oxidised in the body to provide energy for tissue activity and for the maintenance of body temperature. They are a concentrated source of energy, providing 37 kJ (9 kcal) per gram, compared with 16 kJ per gram from carbohydrate and 17 kJ per gram from protein. A sufficiency of energy from carbohydrate and fat ensures that protein is available for tissue formation and repair.

2. Incorporated into body structure. Some fat enters the body cells and constitutes an essential part of their structure.

3. Protection. The deposits of fatty tissue around the vital organs hold these organs in position and protect them from injury.

4. Insulation. Subcutaneous fat prevents loss of heat from the body.

5. Satiety. The presence of fat in the chyme as it passes into the duodenum results in inhibition of gastric peristalsis and acid secretion, thus delaying the emptying time of the stomach and preventing early recurrence of hunger after a meal.

6. Fat-soluble vitamins. The fats of the diet provide the fat-soluble vitamins and assist in their absorption from the intestine.

Fat stores

The chief stores of fatty tissue are under the skin and around the abdominal organs and these are sometimes referred to as the fat depots. Large amounts of fat can be stored in this way. These fat stores are not inert, but are continually being interchanged with the fats circulating in the blood stream, and mobilised for use as fuel.

The metabolism of an unusually large proportion of fat may give rise to ketosis (p. 11). This might occur as a result of a diet very low in carbohydrate, and is a feature of diabetes mellitus where carbohydrate metabolism is impaired through lack of insulin.

Daily intake

Fats have a higher energy value weight for weight than carbohydrate, protein or alcohol. They contribute an important part of the energy content of the diet and improve its palatability.

In the United Kingdom individual fat intakes might be said to range between 80 and 160 g daily. It is not known whether any definite amount of fat is necessary for the maintenance of health.

Ingestion of fat beyond the energy needs of the body leads to deposition of fat in the adipose tissues and contributes to the development of obesity.

ESSENTIAL FATTY ACIDS

Certain highly unsaturated (polyunsaturated) fatty acids are needed by the body and have become known as the essential fatty acids. The essential fatty acids are linoleic, linolenic and arachidonic, the most important of which is linolenic.

Deficiency has not been reported in healthy persons eating a normal diet, but there are indications that it can occur in special circumstances, for example in conjunction with malabsorption of fats, and in persons who have been fed intravenously for a prolonged time without fat being included. There is a connection between the proportion of essential fatty acids in the diet and the incidence of coronary artery disease, and linoleic acid is an important component of the unsaturated fats (e.g. corn oil) included in the special diet sometimes advocated for people prone to this condition.

Vitamin E is important in preventing oxidation of essential fatty acids in the body, thus preserving their chemical structure.

CHOLESTEROL

Cholesterol is a substance usually considered along with the fats. It is synthesised in the body and is also obtained from the diet. It occurs in association with animal tissues and in the United Kingdom the principal dietary source is egg yolk.

Cholesterol is excreted from the body in the bile, where it is held in solution by combining with bile salts. If it is precipitated out of solution it appears in solid form as gall-stones.

PHOSPHOLIPIDS

Phospholipids are substances allied to the fats. Much of the fatty material which constitutes an integral part of body cells is in the form of phospholipids, which are present in large amount in brain and nervous tissue. They are formed as an intermediate stage in fat metabolism and are present in blood plasma.

LIPOPROTEINS

Fats, cholesterol, phospholipids and fatty acids are insoluble in water, but in blood plasma they form soluble combinations with some of the plasma proteins, and in this form they are known as lipoproteins.

QUESTIONS

1. Which foods contain fat?
2. How is fat digested?
3. How do saturated and polyunsaturated fats differ?

4

Proteins

SUMMARY

Proteins are vital constituents of all cells. They are complex structures made from amino acids.

Foods of animal and plant origin both contain proteins. They are hydrolysed by proteolytic enzymes to release amino acids before they are absorbed. An adequate supply of all amino acids is necessary for body growth and repair. Some amino acids can be manufactured by the body. Those which the body cannot synthesise must be provided by the diet and are called essential amino acids.

When carbohydrate intake is restricted, proteins are catabolised to provide energy.

Every living cell has protein as one of its principal constituents. In structure, proteins resemble chains consisting of amino acids linked together. Animals can synthesise proteins from amino acids but are unable to synthesise amino acids. Plants are able to synthesise amino acids from carbon dioxide, water and nitrogen-containing materials from the soil. Thus, man only obtains protein by eating plants or other animals.

Proteins are composed of carbon, hydrogen, oxygen and nitrogen. In some cases mineral elements such as sulphur, phosphorus, iodine and iron and also present. The proteins of the diet are the body's only source of nitrogen.

Very large protein molecules contain many thousands of amino acids, whereas small proteins such as insulin contain less than one hundred. Structurally they are divided into two types depending on the shape of the molecule: fibrous, where the chain remains in its extended form, and globular, where the chain is folded to form an irregularly shaped bulky molecule.

There are thousands of different plant and animal proteins, the exact structure of many is still unknown. All are hydrolysed to amino acids in varying proportions. Examples of protein found in food:

> myosin
> albumin
> casein
> vitellin
> globulin
> gluten

The amino acid content and sequence shows a species variation. Thus, the myosin in beef is different to the myosin in lamb.

Essential amino acids

The human body requires amino acids for making the specific proteins required by its many specialised tissues. Some amino acids it can make itself by converting one to another. This occurs in the liver by a process known as transamination. Those amino acids which the body is either unable to make, or unable to make in sufficient quantities, are called essential amino acids and are listed below.

> histidine
> lysine
> methionine
> valine
> leucine

isoleucine
tryptophan
phenylalanine
threonine

Biological value of proteins

If the diet contains adequate supplies of all the essential amino acids, proteins can be synthesised. If, however, it contains an inadequate amount of one of these proteins, synthesis cannot occur. Protein foods which contain all the essential amino acids in the proportions required by man are said to have a high biological value. Examples of foods with a high biological value are breast milk and hens' eggs.

Limiting amino acids

Protein foods from plant sources tend to have a lower biological value than animal protein foods. The essential amino acids that they lack, or only supply in small amounts, are called the limiting amino acids. Not all foods have the same limiting amino acid, e.g.

Food	Limiting amino acid
wheat	lysine
soya beans	methionine
maize	tryptophan

Supplementary actions of proteins

The lack of an essential amino acid in a food can be overcome by eating, at the same time, another protein food which contains that amino acid. For example, a meal containing wheat as the only protein source lacks lysine and so has a low biological value, as does a meal of beans only, for although they are a rich source of lysine they contain very little methionine. However, a meal which contains both soya beans and wheat has adequate supplies of both lysine and methionine. This fact is of great importance to strict vegetarians who derive their protein entirely from vegetable sources. They require to eat an adequate amount and variety of the foods containing incomplete proteins to ensure a sufficiency of the essential amino acids.

In many parts of the world the staple diet consists largely or entirely of foods of vegetable origin, containing only incomplete proteins. Efforts are at present being made to increase the nutritive value of these diets by the addition of foods which can be produced locally, and which supply the essential amino acids lacking in those already consumed. Some products which have proved of value in this respect are groundnuts (peanuts), soy beans and cotton-seed.

In a mixed diet such as that normally eaten in the United Kingdom the protein is derived from foods of both groups. Approximate protein values for some food portions are given on page 24.

Functions

Proteins are essential constituents of all body tissues.

1. They replace the protein lost during normal metabolism and normal wear and tear. Protein is lost in the formation of hair and nails and as dead cells from the surface of skin and the alimentary tract and in digestive secretions.

2. They produce new tissue. New tissue is formed during periods of growth, recovery from injury, pregnancy and lactation.

3. They are needed in the manufacture of new proteins which perform specific functions in the body—enzymes, hormones and haemoglobin.

4. Protein can be used as an energy source.

Nitrogen balance

It is known that 1 g nitrogen is contained in approximately 6 g protein, the exact figure depending upon the nature and source of the protein. It is thus possible to calculate the nitrogen value of the diet from its protein content. A person is said to be in nitrogen balance when the intake of nitrogen in the diet is equal to the output in urine and faeces and from the skin (normal loss on an adequate diet is 14 g nitrogen but is lower on a poor diet).

Positive nitrogen balance—nitrogen intake exceeds nitrogen loss, so it can be assumed that new tissue is being formed, e.g. growth.

Negative nitrogen balance—nitrogen loss exceeds nitrogen intake, so it can be assumed that tissue is being broken down, e.g. burns, starvation.

Nitrogen balance studies are sometimes performed in order to obtain information about protein requirements, or to assist in the diagnosis of disease.

Digestion, absorption and disposal

Proteins are hydrolysed to amino acids and peptides by digestion. Digestion starts in the stomach where the combination of an acid pH and proteolytic enzymes hydrolyse the proteins to large polypeptides which enter the duodenum. These polypeptides are further hydrolysed by pancreatic proteolytic enzymes to peptides and amino acids. Proteolytic enzymes are secreted in an inactive form that is activated by another enzyme. The amino acids and peptides produced enter the intestinal cells and from there have three fates:

1. They enter the circulating body amino acid pool from which they are built into the structural proteins and specific enzymes which are needed by each cell.

2. They are converted to other amino acids.

3. They are oxidised to produce energy; in some cases the amino acids are converted to glucose first. The urea formed is excreted by the kidneys.

Daily intake

The Committee on Medical Aspects of Food Policy, reporting in 1979, recommended average daily intakes of protein for the United Kingdom. These are reproduced in Appendix 2. It will be seen that for adults they vary between 42 and 84 g daily and represent 10 per cent of the recommended energy intake.

In their deliberations the members of the panel considered firstly minimum protein requirements. They found it necessary, however, to recommend intakes higher than the minimum in order to allow for a palatable diet. They also

Table 4.1 These figures are approximate and for the purpose of comparison only. For more precise information on the composition of foods, Appendix 4 should be consulted.

	Protein (g)
50 g egg (1 egg)	6
30 g cheese	6
50 g cottage cheese	7
200 ml milk (1 glass)	6
60 g fish cooked	12
50 g meat cooked	12
30 g bread (1 slice toasting pan)	2
30 g biscuit or cake	2
30 g cereal (e.g. flour, oatmeal, rice, semolina, cornflakes)	2
100 g (3 tablesp.) cabbage or carrot boiled	1
180 g potato boiled (1 medium size)	3
50 g butter beans boiled (2 tablesp.)	3
50 g peas or beans boiled	2
100 g baked beans in tomato sauce (2 tablesp.)	5
15 g peanut butter (2 teasp.)	3
200 g lentil soup (1 serving) home made	9
200 g vegetable soup canned	3
1 slice toast and a serving of baked beans in tomato sauce	8
1 slice bread spread with 2 teasp. peanut butter	6

considered other important nutrients such as B complex vitamins which are found in association with protein in foods. The final figures are therefore intended to be used as a guide in the planning and assessment of diets and should not be applied to the protein requirements of individuals.

It is advisable that some protein should be derived from foods of animal origin—milk, eggs, cheese, fish and meat—which are best able to supply the essential amino acids. It should be remembered also that the value of these foods is partly determined by the relatively high contribution they make towards the intake of other essential nutrients.

The Table 4.1 gives the approximate protein content of some average food portions.

Insufficient protein intake

It is most unusual in this country to meet with obvious signs of protein deficiency resulting from grossly defective diet, but it is not known to what extent minor deficiencies may arise, and may be responsible for ill-health and impaired development. Marginal intakes should be avoided, especially in times of increased need such as growth, pregnancy, lactation, and during recovery from injury, when insufficient protein can impair wound healing and increase susceptibility to infection.

Protein deficiency may arise as a result of illness.

1. If the energy requirement is increased, as in fevers or hyperthyroidism, the use of protein for energy production may result in a lack of protein for growth and replacement, and this may be aggravated by the withdrawal of protein from the body tissues to help meet energy needs.

2. Burns, fractures and other injuries, including those resulting from operative procedures, are followed by a period when breakdown of body protein exceeds intake, in other words a period of negative nitrogen balance.

3. Deficiency may also result from failure to utilise protein, as occurs in some disorders affecting the gastrointestinal tract, and when the liver is diseased.

4. Protein deficiency may be the result of excessive loss of protein from the body, as occurs in some kidney disorders, as a result of harmorrhage, and in the fluid which exudes from burned surfaces.

Protein energy malnutrition (PEM)

Protein energy malnutrition is the general term used to describe the spectrum of illnesses caused by an inadequate diet, deficient in protein and often in energy too, that occurs mainly in developing countries. There are two extreme forms:

Kwashiorkor due to a dietary deficiency of protein.

Marasmus due to dietary deficiencies of both protein and energy.

In practice the clinical picture is usually mixed and is often complicated by other specific vitamin and mineral deficiencies, for example vitamin A and iron.

Kwashiorkor

In rural areas this is the form of PEM that predominates. It develops during early childhood when, after prolonged breast feeding, the child is weaned onto a diet based on a starchy staple food which has a low protein content. Although able to eat sufficient to satisfy his energy requirements, this quantity of food does not contain adequate protein. Children whose diet is deficient in protein are unable to synthesise sufficient new body proteins. This results in retardation of growth, increased susceptibility to infection and slow recovery from injury and infection. Some physiological adaptation to a low protein intake does occur but any condition which increases protein requirement, injury or infection, can precipitate severe Kwashiorkor. Its clinical signs are growth retardation, oedema, muscle wasting, liver enlargement, skin and hair pigmentation changes.

Marasmus

Unlike Kwashiorkor, this is more common in urban areas. Its incidence there is increasing, particularly amongst those who have recently moved from rural areas. Marasmus develops when the diet lacks sufficient energy and protein. It is sometimes referred to as childhood starvation and is most commonly caused by incorrect bottle feeding. The milk is over diluted and so provides an inadequate diet. Gastroenteritis is common and may precipitate marasmus by increasing intestinal losses and nutritional requirements and also because it is often treated with starvation by the parents. Its clinical signs are:

> muscle wasting
> loss of sub-cutaneous fat layer
> growth retardation.

PEM also occurs in adults though it is generally less severe because the relative protein requirement is lower. It results in small stature and low weight, high disease prevalence, a shorter life expectancy and low birth weight in the babies of marasmic mothers.

PEM is a major problem that confronts developing countries and can be overcome by the following public health measures:

Breast feeding should be encouraged. Bottle feeding is unsatisfactory both because of its cost and the need for sterilisation and for clean water. However, it must be remembered that the nutritional requirements of the mother are increased whilst she is breast feeding. A combination of poor maternal diet and prolonged breast feeding can cause Kwashiorkor.

Nutritional supplements are needed for vulnerable groups. Children, pregnant and lactating women, whose nutritional needs are not met by their diet.

Nutrition education

This must be specific to the community and is most successfully carried out in maternal and child health centres where mothers can learn of the need for an adequate diet and how to provide it.

Improved sanitary conditions and provision of clean water will reduce the incidence of infections disease, particularly gastroenteritis.

QUESTIONS

1. Why is it important to include a wide variety of protein sources in the diet?
2. How is protein utilised by the body?
3. What is meant by nitrogen balance?

5

Mineral elements and water

SUMMARY

The body cannot synthesise minerals, they have to be provided by the diet. Most minerals can be detected in the body, those that are only required in minute amounts are called trace elements.

Mineral elements are incorporated into the bones and teeth and proteins. They are essential for the normal functioning of some enzymes and are important in controlling the composition of the body fluids.

About 65 per cent of the body weight is water. This is the most important of all nutrients and is contained in solid food as well as in drinks. A small amount is produced by metabolism. Water is the medium in which almost all metabolic processes occur. Water is lost in the breath as well as in sweat, urine and faeces. Man can live for weeks without food, but only for days without water.

Mineral elements comprise only 3 per cent approximately of the total body weight. Their presence is, however, of vital importance. They are essential constituents of the soft tissues, fluids and skeleton, the latter containing a large proportion

28

of the body's mineral content. Some minerals known to be concerned in body processes are listed below

calcium	iron	manganese
phosphorus	fluorine	magnesium
potassium	copper	chromium
sulphur	zinc	selenium
sodium	iodine	
chlorine	cobalt	

Many of the minerals in foods are in the form of salts and salts are present in all the tissues and fluids of the body. Minerals in the body have three functions:

1. They are constituents of bones and teeth, giving them their strength and rigidity, e.g.,calcium, phosphorus and magnesium.

2. They form soluble salts and so control the composition of body fluids. Sodium and chloride are important in the extracellular fluid and blood; potassium, magnesium and phosphorus are important in the intracellular fluid.

3. They are incorporated into enzymes and proteins. Sulphur is part of the amino acids, methionine and cysteine.

CALCIUM

Of all the minerals in the body calcium occurs in the greatest amount. The body of a well-nourished adult contains 1–1.5 kg calcium, 90 per cent of which is found in the bones and teeth in the form of a complex salt. Deposits of this salt in the original soft bone matrix give the necessary rigidity, and in the case of teeth contribute to hardness and resistance to decay. The small amount of calcium in the tissue fluids plays a part in controlling the action of heart and skeletal muscle and the excitability of nerves. Calcium also functions in the clotting of blood.

Absorption and utilisation

Where the type of diet normally consumed by Western peoples is concerned, it has been estimated that only 20 to 30 per cent of the calcium is absorbed from the alimentary tract.

The factors affecting the absorption of calcium are only partially understood.

* Vitamin D is concerned in both the absorption of calcium from the gut and its deposition in bone. In the absence of sufficient of the vitamin these processes are seriously impaired.

Absorption is also affected by other constituents of the diet. Proteins have a favourable effect on calcium absorption because soluble salts which can be easily absorbed are formed between calcium and amino acids. Wholemeal cereal products and some fruits and vegetables reduce calcium absorption. The phytic acid occurring in cereals and the oxalic acid occurring in vegetables and fruit combine with calcium to form insoluble salts which cannot be absorbed. Yeast contains the enzyme phytase which destroys the phytic acid. Diets containing a lot of whole grain cereal are only likely to cause calcium deficiency if the cereal is eaten in an unleavened form such as chapattis.

Dietary sources

Milk has a high content of available calcium, is palatable, inexpensive and a staple food. Cheese also has a high calcium content. Two thirds of the calcium content of the British diet is provided by dairy produce. Flour, with the exception of wholemeal, is fortified with calcium with the result that bread and similar foods made from fortified flour are of value as a source of this mineral. In the United Kingdom most of the calcium of the diet comes from these foods. Others containing useful supplementary amounts are eggs, fish such as salmon and sardines of which the small bones are eaten, cabbage and broccoli. Dried milk is a concentrated source of calcium. A significant amount may be obtained from hard water, which can contain up to 50 mg per litre.

Dietary requirements

Calcium is excreted in the urine and faeces and dietary calcium is required to make good these losses. Additional amounts are needed—for growth throughout childhood and adolescence, during pregnancy to meet the requirements of the fetus, and during lactation for secretion in the milk which supplies the calcium needed by the growing infant. The Committee on Medical Aspects of Food Policy recommended a dietary intake of 500 mg daily for adults, increasing to 1200 mg in the third trimester of pregnancy and in lactation. Further details are given in Appendix 2. These recommendations are not intended to be a statement of calcium requirements, about which more requires to be known. Half a litre of milk supplies approximately 500 mg calcium. The value of milk as a source of this mineral is therefore apparent.

Deficiency

Calcium may be lacking in the body if absorption is impaired as in the malabsorption syndrome or as a result of lack of vitamin D. A diet low in available calcium may be a contributing factor. Deficiency of calcium in the body gives rise to the development of rickets in childhood and osteomalacia in adult life. These conditions are discussed further in the section on vitamin D. ②Tetani - spasm of muscle
③Bleeding tendencies

PHOSPHORUS

Phosphorus comes next to calcium in the amount present in the body. The greater part of body phosphorus is combined with calcium in the bones and teeth. It is also necessary for the formation of essential cell components (the phospholipids), plays a part in the release of energy from carbohydrate and fat, assists absorption of carbohydrate from the small intestine and helps to maintain acid/base balance in the body fluids.

Absorption

As in the case of calcium, absorption depends upon the formation of soluble salts. Excessive use of antacids containing magnesium and aluminium can limit phosphorus absorption by the formation of insoluble salts.

Dietary sources

Phosphorus is widely distributed in foods. In general, meat, fish, milk, cheese, eggs and cereals contain more phosphorus than vegetables and fruits.

Deficiency

Dietary deficiency is unlikely to occur. The foods upon which we depend for much of our calcium have a high phosphorus content, and it may be said that an adequacy of calcium ensures also a sufficiency of phosphorus. However, it can occur in alcoholics, patients with renal disease and patients receiving total parenteral nutrition.

IRON

The total iron content of the body is quite small, and in the case of a man of average size is estimated to be about 4 g.

Iron is necessary for the formation of haemoglobin, a constituent of the red blood cells. Haemoglobin is responsible for the transport of oxygen and carbon dioxide between the lungs and the tissues, and is the pigment which gives the blood its red colour. Iron is found in the muscle pigment myoglobin; it is also an important constituent of many enzyme systems. 0.5–1 g of iron is stored as ferritin in the liver, spleen and bone marrow. This iron is used to restore the haemoglobin level to normal after haemorrhage.

Absorption

The greater part of the iron in food is not absorbed by the body.

The factors affecting absorption are not fully understood. The presence of other dietary constituents plays a part. Iron is more readily absorbed from some sources, e.g. meat, than others and some foods interact with each other to aid iron absorption whilst others inhibit it, for example, absorption is facilitated by the presence of ascorbic acid and inhibited by the phytic acid which is present in whole grain cereals.

Vit. C (Absorbic acid assists in absorption of iron).

There is an association between iron absorption and the presence of the hydrochloric acid and enzymes of the gastric juice, and absorption is reduced in persons with a lack of gastric secretion.

The passage of iron through the intestinal mucosa is regulated in such a way that iron is only absorbed when required, any dietary excess appearing in the faeces.

Food sources

Most of the iron of the average diet is derived from eggs, meat, fish, flour, bread and vegetables, especially the green leafy vegetables. These foods, which are moderate in iron content, contribute valuable amounts, as they are eaten regularly. Liver has a high content of iron. Treacle, and dried fruits such as raisins, prunes and apricots, contain considerable amounts. More requires to be known about the relative availability to the body of iron present in different foods. Two types of iron are found in foods: fresh foods contain haem iron (that is, iron in haemoglobin), and fruit and vegetables contain iron as ferric complexes.

Dietary requirement

1. To make good the very small amount which is constantly lost to the body, principally in the urine.
2. To replace loss due to menstruation.
3. For the formation of new haemoglobin in pregnancy, childhood and adolescence.
4. In lactation for secretion in the milk.
5. To make good loss of iron due to bleeding.

The Committee on Medical Aspects of Food Policy stressed the difficulties of deciding upon desirable intake levels in view of the many variables, for example the factors affecting absorption. They nevertheless thought it advisable to give some guidance and suggested 10 mg daily for men and post-menopausal women, 12 mg for menstruating women, 13 mg during pregnancy and 15 mg in lactation. Further figures are given in Appendix 2.

Deficiency

Inadequate iron for red cell formation results in iron-deficiency anaemia. This condition is further discussed in Chapter 27.

IODINE

The trace element iodine is a constituent of thyroxine, the hormone secreted by the thyroid gland. Thyroxine controls the rate of tissue activity, or metabolic rate, and is vital to physical and mental development.

Dietary sources

Iodine is present in very small amount in many foods, the best sources being vegetables and sea fish.

The iodine content of agricultural produce depends upon the amount of iodine in the soil in the district where the food was produced rather than on the nature of the food itself. Soils vary greatly in iodine content, some containing very little.

Goitrogens

Some foods have been found to contain substances which interfere with the utilisation of iodine. These substances are known as goitrogens. Cabbage and turnip contain goitrogenic material. There is evidence to suggest that water may have goitrogenic properties when contaminated with faeces, and that some hard waters are goitrogenic.

Iodine deficiency

Iodine deficiency is prevalent in communities where dietary intake is low, or insufficient to counteract the effect of goitrogenic factors operating in the particular area. The Goitre Sub-Committee of the Medical Research Council has recommended that potassium iodide be added to common salt as a means of reducing the incidence of iodine deficiency in Great Britain. To date this recommendation has not been adopted. Iodised salt, however, is available on demand. Programmes of supplementation on a community scale have been adopted with good results in many other countries, including the United States, Switzerland, Australia and New Zealand.

Effects of iodine deficiency

If sufficient iodine is not available for formation of thyroxine the thyroid gland enlarges in an effort to maintain its normal output of the hormone, and gives rise to a swelling of the neck. This condition is known as endemic goitre. The word 'endemic' means 'commonly found in certain populations'.

Deficiency of iodine during pregnancy and infancy results in a failure of physical and mental development of the child, a condition sometimes known as cretinism.

Iodine deficiency is found in certain parts of the United Kingdom, for example in Derbyshire.

FLUORINE

The body contains traces of fluorine, principally in the teeth and the skeleton. This mineral is present in water, which, although containing only minute amounts, is the chief dietary source. Traces are also present in many foods.

Interest in fluorine where human nutrition is concerned centres around its association with the prevention of dental caries. It has been shown that in districts where fluorine is present in water to the extent of 1 part per million, teeth are more resistant to decay than in districts where the water contains smaller amounts. To bring about this effect the fluorine must be available while calcification is taking place rather than after the teeth have already matured. If the fluorine content of the water is in excess of this amount permanent chalk-white mottling appears on the teeth in a proportion of cases. Higher concentrations result in an increase in the proportion of cases of mottling and in the mottling taking on a permanent brown discoloration.

This has raised the question of whether or not public water supplies which are deficient in fluorine should have this mineral added to the level required for maximum prevention of dental caries, and yet not high enough to cause discoloration. Studies in the United States have shown that children living in areas where the drinking water contains 1 part per million or more of fluorine, show an incidence of dental caries up to 60 per cent less than in areas where the water is deficient in this mineral. It has also been shown that a comparable effect may be obtained by artificial flouridation of water supplies which are low in fluorine content. Trials carried out in this country have furnished similar evidence of the benefits of the protective level of fluorine in drinking water. Artificial fluoridation of water supplies is being carried out extensively in the United States and has been introduced in many other countries, including the United Kingdom.

SODIUM

Physiological functions of sodium

The body sodium is found principally in the blood plasma and the fluid surrounding the tissues. It plays an important part in the production of the osmotic pressure which regulates fluid exchanges between the cells and the surrounding tissue fluid. The amount of sodium in extracellular fluid determines its volume.

Dietary sources

Most of the sodium of the diet comes from sodium chloride (common salt) which is used as a condiment in cooking and at the table, and for the preservation of such foods as cheese, ham, tongue, fish and vegetables. Sodium also occurs as a natural constituent of foods. On the whole, milk, cheese, eggs, meat and fish have a higher sodium content than fruits, vegetables and cereals. Vegetables with a high sodium content include spinach and celery.

Dietary requirement

Sufficient sodium is present in foods to ensure an adequacy

of this mineral, and the body can adjust itself to wide variations in intake by excreting any excess in the urine. In certain diseases, however, sodium is retained in the body in excessive amounts, and in these circumstances it may be necessary to restrict dietary intake. There is evidence linking hypertension with a high salt intake, so it is advisable to discourage a high salt intake.

Hypernatraemia - high sodium (N.A)
Hyponatraemia - low sodium (N.A)

Deficiency

Sodium is excreted principally in urine and in sweat. Normally the sodium content of the body is maintained by the kidneys at an almost constant level. If sweating is very profuse, however, as occurs in hot climates, sodium depletion can occur. This gives rise to symptoms which include excessive fatigue and muscle cramps. These symptoms are also experienced by people whose occupations involve working in extremely hot surroundings. The condition may be remedied, or its occurrence prevented, by an increased salt intake.

In temperate climates such as that of the British Isles sodium depletion due to excessive sweating is not likely to occur, except as an occupational hazard, but loss of sodium is seen in conjunction with certain pathological conditions which include severe and prolonged vomiting and diarrhoea, loss of exudate from burns, and Addison's disease (the result of under-activity of the suprarenal glands).

POTASSIUM

Hypokalaemia (K) a low amount of Potassium in blood stream

Potassium is present principally in body cells. Its action complements that of sodium. Normally the kidneys play an important part in regulating the potassium content of the body. Excessive retention occurs in association with some kidney disorders and also in Addison's disease, and brings about cardiac arrest. Deficiency can result from prolonged vomiting or diarrhoea, or as a result of oral diuretic therapy, and causes muscle paralysis. The possibility of a dietary deficiency occurring is remote. Fruit and vegetables are rich sources of potassium.

Hyperkalaemia (K) a high potassium in blood stream.

Normal 3.5 - 4.5 milimoles per litre

CHLORINE

Chlorine is obtained from sodium chloride and is also present in most foods. Depletion can result from prolonged vomiting, but inadequate intake is not likely to occur.

MAGNESIUM

Magnesium is another essential element unlikely to be lacking in the diet. Deficiency, however, sometimes occurs along with other metabolic disturbances in certain diseases, for example chronic malabsorption, severe diarrhoea, chronic renal failure, chronic alcoholism, and protein-energy malnutrition. It has also been known to occur following surgical removal of the parathyroid glands and in conjunction with the prolonged use of diuretics.

COPPER

Copper has been found to be necessary along with iron to promote recovery from anaemia in malnourished infants in impoverished communities where feeding has depended upon cow's milk and cereals. Deficiency has occurred during rehabilitation from kwashiorkor and marasmus, if the diets used have been low in copper. Cow's milk has a low copper content. Fruits, Vegs, Red Meat

ZINC

Deficiency of zinc can cause symptoms which include growth failure and impaired healing of wounds. Factors predisposing to deficiency include: diets lacking in zinc in a form readily available to the body, for example containing whole grain cereals which can interfere with zinc absorption; parasites causing chronic blood loss; excessive sweating due to high environmental temperature; malabsorption of food; surgery;

Hypog

burns. Simple dietary deficiency appears to be uncommon in Western communities.

Sources :- same as calcium

COBALT

Cobalt is the constituent of vitamin B_{12}, which is necessary for normal development of red blood cells.

Other minerals are present, some in trace amounts, in human tissues, examples are cadmium and selenium. Some of these are essential but in many cases their function is poorly understood. As they are not likely to be lacking in the diet, and as no deficiency states have been reported, they do not require consideration from a nutritional point of view.

WATER

Water constitutes about 65 to 70 per cent of the total body weight and is the medium in which almost every body process takes place. When one considers some of the many ways in which it promotes the functions of the body its importance becomes apparent.

Water is the basis of intracellular and extracellular fluids and is a constituent of all the body's secretions and excretions.

The products of digestion are absorbed into the body in a fluid medium and distributed in blood and lymph.

The chemical reactions involved in metabolism also require a fluid medium, and the waste products are conveyed in the blood stream to the kidneys and the lungs for excretion. Sufficient water is required to ensure an adequate urine flow and to facilitate the passage of the faeces along the colon so that constipation does not occur.

The joints are bathed in a lubricating fluid which prevents friction when movement takes place.

Body temperature is largely controlled by evaporation of moisture from the skin and the lungs.

A constant supply of water is essential. Thus people who undergo long fasts can live on their body reserves of protein, fat, carbohydrate and other nutrients for several weeks provided water is available, whereas if it were withheld they would probably die in a few days.

Sources

1. A large part of the water required by the body is supplied by milk, tea, water and other beverages, and such foods as soup.

2. Water is a constituent of most foods, even although they may be solid in consistency. Thus bread contains approximately 36 per cent of water, fish 65 per cent, meat 50 to 70 per cent and vegetables and fruits 80 to 90 per cent.

3. When carbohydrates, fats and proteins are metabolised water is produced. This is known as metabolic water. It is of particular importance to certain forms of animal life. Thus hibernating animals depend during their dormant period on water produced as a result of metabolism.

Water balance

Water is lost from the body in urine, faeces, sweat and in the breath. A sensation of thirst normally ensures an adequate intake. By means of a regulatory mechanism in the kidneys, as a result of which a variable volume of urine is secreted, a balance is maintained between intake and output.

Requirement

An average adult living in a temperate climate requires approximately 2500 ml of water daily. The actual amount he ingests depends both on climate and habit.

Drinks provide 1000–2500 ml
Food provides 1000–1500 ml
Metabolism provides 200–400 ml.

Requirements vary according to the amount lost in sweat and more water is required by people who exercise vigorously, or who work in hot surroundings. As we have already seen, loss of a large volume of sweat necessitates the replacement of salt as well as water.

Water depletion can occur in conditions such as prolonged vomiting and diarrhoea, haemorrhage, extensive burns and in uncontrolled diabetes mellitus. The term dehydration means lack of water, but is often used as implying a lack of certain mineral elements also, particularly sodium.

QUESTIONS

1. Which foods are rich sources of calcium?
2. What is calcium used for?
3. Which foods should a vegetarian eat to prevent iron deficiency anaemia?
4. Why is water such a vital nutrient?

6

✳ Vitamins

SUMMARY

Vitamins are essential for normal nutrition. They are organic substances found in small amounts in a wide variety of foods. They cannot be utilised to supply energy.

Vitamins are divided into two groups:
✳ 1. The fat soluble vitamins—A, D, E and K.
✳ 2. The water soluble vitamins—thiamin, riboflavin, niacin, pyridoxine, folic acid, B_{12} and vitamin C,

The vitamins each have different physiological functions and are not related chemically.

A diet which contains an inadequate amount of a vitamin leads to the development of specific deficiency symptoms.

INTRODUCTION

The term vitamin is a shortened form of vitalamine. This term was first used in 1911 by Casimir Funk to describe a substance that he isolated from rice polishings that both cured and prevented beri-beri in chickens.

One of the earliest records of the cure of a vitamin deficiency disorder, although it was not recognised as such then, was in an Egyptian Medical Treatise of 1500BC where eating roast ox liver was recommended as a treatment for night blindness. During the eighteenth century, Lind cured sailors with scurvy with citrus fruit juice, and, during the nineteenth century, beri-beri was cured in the Japanese navy be adding extra meat and dried milk to the daily rice ration. It was not realised that a specific deficiency was causing the disease and that the food cured this deficiency. At this time the only known nutrients were protein, fat, carbohydrate, mineral elements and water.

A vitamin is an organic substance which an organism must obtain from its environment in minute amounts; it is essential for normal metabolism.

Structure and function

Vitamins have different specific chemical structures and physiological functions. Generally, they act by promoting a specific chemical reaction in a metabolic process. If the vitamin is lacking the metabolic process cannot proceed and the body becomes diseased. When vitamins were first isolated they were identified by a letter of the alphabet. Once their chemical composition was understood they were given an appropriate name, for example vitamin C became ascorbic acid.

Sometimes the vitamin can only be obtained directly from food, for example, ascorbic acid.

In other instances foods also contain a very closely related substance known as the pro-vitamin or vitamin precursor, which can be converted into the vitamin in the body, for example, vitamin A.

Where vitamin D is concerned diet is not the only source as the precursor is manufactured in the body and converted in the skin to the vitamin under the influence of sunlight.

Some vitamins are formed in the intestine by bacteria, and part of the body's requirement may be met in this way. Vitamin K and many of the vitamins of the B group are produced in the intestine as a result of bacterial action. In some cases, however, there is some doubt as to how much of the vitamin formed in this way is absorbed from the digestive tract.

Classification of vitamins

Vitamins may be classified as either fat-soluble or water-soluble:

Fat-soluble	Water soluble
vitamin A	vitamins of the B group
vitamin D	vitamin C
vitamin E	
vitamin K	

Large doses of fat soluble vitamins are harmful because they cannot be excreted and are stored in the body. Water soluble vitamins are excreted in the urine, so large doses are not harmful.

Recommended daily intake

The exact amount of each vitamin needed for optimum health is not known and probably varies greatly from one person to another. The Committee on Medical Aspects of Food Policy, 1979, has made certain recommendations which, it considers, would meet the requirements of average healthy persons. These recommendations are reproduced in Appendix 2.

q. Classify Vits + outline role of Vits in prevention of disease

VITAMIN A (RETINOL) *Fat-soluble vit*

Functions of vitamin A

eyes 1. *Night vision.* Vitamin A is essential for the formation of the retinal pigment Rhodopsin. It is this pigment that enables the eye to see in dim light. This pigment decomposes in the presence of bright light. It is regenerated and requires vitamin A for its regeneration.

skin 2. *Healthy epithelial tissue.* Vitamin A is necessary for maintaining the integrity of epithelial tissue and mucous membranes.

teeth + bone 3. *Normal development of teeth and bones.*

Sources of vitamin A

β carotene is the precursor of vitamin A; it is a yellow pigment which occurs in many plants, particularly those with yellow,

q Name the vit. deficiency diseases

Table 6.1 Vitamin A

Sources
1. Formed in human tissues from plant pigment carotene
2. Formed in tissues of food producing animals and found in milk, eggs, liver and other foods.

Functions
1. Integrity of epithelial tissue
2. Dark-adaptation

Deficiency
1. Night-blindness
2. Mucous membrane infections

red or dark green colouring. Animals, including humans, can convert the carotene of their food into vitamin A. Humans obtain the vitamin partly from animal foods in which it has already been formed and partly from the carotene present in vegetables, fruits and some animal products.

Foods especially rich in carotene include cabbage and lettuce, especially the dark-green leaves; spinach, tomato, carrot, peaches, apricots and prunes.

Preformed vitamin A

The best sources of the already formed vitamin are liver, kidney, egg yolk, milk, butter, cheese, cream, oily fish such as herrings, sardines and salmon, and vitaminised margarine which, although not an animal product, is artificially fortified with the vitamin. Cod and halibut liver oils are particularly rich sources of vitamin A.

Vitamin content of vitamin A

This varies greatly with the diet of the animal concerned. Thus in summer when the cows are out of grass and their diet is high in carotene the vitamin content of milk and its products is at its best.

Effect on vitamin A of cooking and storage of foods

Vitamin A and carotene are not destroyed by most methods

of cooking; some loss occurs at high temperatures, as in frying. Cod and halibut liver oils in containers of clear glass should not be exposed to light, as destruction of vitamin A will result.

Recommended intake

Since vitamin A activity is possessed in different degrees by the vitamin (retinol) itself and by carotene, the Committee on Medical Aspects of Food Policy suggested that vitamin A be measured in retinol equivalents.

They recommended for adults a daily intake of 750 μg retinol recommended rising to 1200 μg during lactation. Further details will be found in Appendix 2.

Until now it has been common practice to measure vitamin A in international units (iu) and carotene in milligrams. 1 μg retinol equivalent is equal to 1 μg retinol, or 3.33 iu of the vitamin, or 6 μg β carotene.

Effects of deficiency

1. Night blindness

The first sign of vitamin A deficiency is impaired ability of the eye to adapt to vision in a dim light. This is known as poor dark adaptation, or night blindness.

2. Deterioration of mucous membrane

A more serious deficiency results in deterioration of mucous membranes, which become dried and hardened, or keratinised. The resultant accumulation of dead cells encourages local infections, for example of the respiratory tract. In some cases the skin becomes dried and the ducts are blocked with dead cells, giving rise to a roughened appearance.

3. Xerophthalmia

Deterioration of the eye occurs, particularly among children. The conjunctiva becomes keratinised, giving rise to xerophthalmia, or dry-eye, and a softening of the cornea—keratomalacia—may take place and may result in infection, ulceration and permanent blindness.

Education in nutrition, the addition of vitamin A to margarine, the routine issue of milk to school children, and vitamin concentrates to infants and to pregnant and nursing mothers, have helped to make deficiency of this vitamin a rare occurrence in the United Kingdom. However, deficiency still occurs in India, Africa, Ceylon and other Eastern countries, and is the cause of much preventable blindness among children.

VITAMIN D (CALCIFEROL)

Functions of vitamin D

Vitamin D facilitates the absorption of calcium from the small intestine and the calcification of the skeleton.

Vitamin D formation

The precursors of vitamin D belong to a group of substances known as sterols. They are converted to vitamin D on exposure to ultra-violet light. Animals manufacture the vitamin from 7-dehydrocholesterol, a sterol which is present in animal fats, and which is converted to vitamin D on exposure to the ultra-violet rays of sunlight. In humans the vitamin is formed on or near the surface of the skin. It is interesting to note that some mammals are thought to obtain the vitamin by licking their fur; in the case of birds the vitamin precursor is present in the oil of the preen gland, which is spread over the feathers by the bird and becomes irradiated, the vitamin being subsequently either directly absorbed or ingested during preening.

Vitamin D may also be produced by the irradiation of a plant sterol which is present in yeasts and fungi. This form of the vitamin is prepared commercially and used in medicinal preparations and for the fortification of such foods as margarine. It is known as vitamin D_2 or ergocalciferol, while the vitamin is present in animal tissues is known as vitamin D_3 or cholecalciferol. These two appear to be of equal potency for man.

Table 6.2 Vitamin D

Sources
1. Action of *ultra-violet light* on skin
2. Already present in *certain foods of animal origin*, e.g., oily fish, eggs
3. Prepared *artificially* by irradiation of a plant sterol, and used in *medicinal preparations, vitaminised margarine, etc.*

Functions
Promotes *absorption of calcium* from small bowel and *deposition in bone*

Deficiency
Rickets
Osteomalacia

Sources of vitamin D

1. Non-dietary

We have seen that humans obtain vitamin D as a result of exposure of the skin to the ultra-violet rays of sunlight.

2. Dietary

Vitamin D is also present in foods of animal origin in which it has already been formed, and is found in eggs, butter and oily fish such as herrings, sardines and salmon. Cod and halibut liver oils are particularly rich sources. Margarine is artificially fortified with the vitamin. It might be expected that milk and cheese would be good sources of vitamin D, but in fact they contain only small amounts. Proprietary milks used for feeding babies, also the fortified infant cereal foods, are in many cases almost the only vitamin D-containing components of the diet for this age group.

Fortification of dairy produce

Both vitamins A and D are removed with the fat from milk during the skimming process. Any vitamin A or D in products made from skimmed milk has to be added.

Effect of cooking, storage and preservation

Vitamin D is not affected by storage, preservation or cooking of food.

Recommended intake

Very little information is available on which to base an estimation of vitamin D requirements. It is possible that for adults no dietary intake is necessary provided there is adequate exposure to sunlight. This is not always the case in this country. Children and adolescents during the winter may possibly lack adequate vitamin D. Those who are partially or totally housebound certainly require a dietary source, or alternatively a supplement of the vitamin. Some recommendations will be found in Appendix 2.

Deficiency

Deficiency of vitamin D leads to rickets in young children and osteomalacia in adults.

Rickets

In rickets the calcification of the skeleton is impaired. The bones remain stunted and soft and the weight of the child and the pull of the muscles give rise to deformities such as bow legs, narrowing of the pelvis, curvature of the spine and undue prominence of the sternum known as pigeon chest. Failure of calcification leads to accumulation of cartilage at the ends of the long bones. This results in swellings which are particularly apparent at the wrists and ankles. Beading of the ribs, called the rachitic rosary, results from accumulation of cartilage at the junctions of cartilage and ribs. Development of teeth may be delayed. Bossing of the skull may result in the development of a square-shaped head, and the closure of the anterior fontanelle may be delayed. The child is restless and excessive perspiration occurs, especially of the head. There is impaired muscle tone, giving rise to a pot-bellied appearance. Gastrointestinal upsets occur.

✳ Osteomalacia

Osteomalacia in adults corresponds to rickets in children. In some countries it is a complication of pregnancy, when vitamin D requirements are increased to meet the needs of the mother and the fetus. If these requirements are not met the skeleton of the mother becomes demineralised. Bone deformities and fractures occur, and deformity of the pelvis may make normal delivery of the child impossible.

In both rickets and osteomalacia a low blood calcium level may give rise to a form of muscle spasm known as tetany.

Incidence of rickets and osteomalacia

Vitamin D is present in foods of the normal diet in comparatively small amounts which vary with the extent to which the animal has been exposed to sunlight, and naturally occurring foods cannot be depended upon as a source of supply. The action of the ultra-violet rays of sunlight cannot be depended upon either as they are impeded by cloud, atmospheric dust, window glass and clothing.

Rickets is known to have been of frequent occurrence in the United Kingdom for some hundreds of years. It has been particularly prevalent among the poor of large cities who could not afford to feed their children adequately, and who did not benefit from the effect of sunlight because of poor social conditions and the prevalence of cloud and smoke.

Since the discovery in the 1920s of vitamin D and its anti-rachitic effect much has been done to improve this state of affairs. Improved standards of living, education in nutrition, the routine administration of vitamin concentrates to infants and pregnant and nursing mothers, and the addition of vitamin D to margarine and to the dried and evaporated milks and cereal foods used in infant feeding, have combined to make rickets uncommon among British children. It cannot, however, be considered entirely a thing of the past, and in recent years it has become a serious health problem among Indian and Pakistani immigrants to Great Britain. The dietary problems of immigrants are discussed in Chapter 15.

Low vitamin D intake probably contributes to the development of osteomalacia which has been reported among elderly women in the United Kingdom. Recently, osteomalacia has been encountered among immigrants from India and Pakistan. Osteomalacia in its most serious form occurs in some Eastern countries, where the diet is lacking in calcium and vitamin D and where there is very little sunshine. It occurs also in women who are never exposed to the sun, for example among those living under the purdah system.

VITAMIN E (tocopherol)

Functions

Vitamin E has been shown to be necessary for some animal species. Most of the experimental work has been done on rats, in which deficiency of this vitamin causes failure of reproduction. The function of vitamin E in the human body is not fully understood. There is however evidence to suggest that it plays a part in processes controlling oxidation in body tissues. Deficiency is unknown under normal conditions.

Vit E present in soaps + beauty products etc) - has not been proven

Sources

This vitamin is widely distributed in foods. Wheat germ and wheat germ oil are particularly rich sources. It is also present in the germinating part of other seeds and in green leafy vegetables. Other foods contain smaller amounts.

VITAMIN K

Function

Vitamin K is known as the anti-haemorrhagic vitamin as it maintains in the blood normal levels of prothrombin and other factors necessary for blood clotting.

Sources

Many foods contain vitamin K, green vegetables being particularly rich sources. It is thought that humans obtain this vitamin as a result of production by bacteria in the intestine.

Requirement

Vitamin K requirement is believed to be very small and easily met by bacterial synthesis and dietary intake.

Deficiency

When deficiency of vitamin K is observed it is usually due to a failure of absorption of the vitamin from the alimentary tract, often accompanying impaired fat absorption, e.g., in disease of the small bowel.

In newly born infants a fall occurs, in the first few days of life, in the vitamin K-dependent blood coagulation factors, of which prothrombin is one, and is occasionally associated with bleeding, for example from the cord, or into the gastrointestinal tract. Administration of vitamin K is effective in some cases of neonatal bleeding and it is thought that the low dietary intake of this vitamin during the first few days of life, and the fact that the bacteria responsible for synthesis of the vitamin have not yet become established in the intestine, may be factors contributing to its development. Vitamin K is given routinely to infants who have had an instrumental delivery, for example with the aid of forceps, or who show signs of haemorrhage. Some physicians give vitamin K routinely to all infants at birth.

Usually given in form of Konakeon – Vit K₁
Konakeon.

ABSORPTION OF FAT-SOLUBLE VITAMINS

Absorption of the fat-soluble vitamins is associated with the simultaneous absorption of fat and is assisted by the emulsifying action of bile. A deficiency of these vitamins can occur when excessive amounts of fat escape digestion and absorption and are excreted in the faeces. Such disturbances have been known to induce rickets and osteomalacia.

In obstructive jaundice, when bile is prevented from entering the duodenum, poor absorption of vitamin K can result in serious haemorrhage during operation to remove the obstruction. The administration of the vitamin by injection before the operation eliminates this risk.

Fat-soluble vitamins are also soluble in mineral oils, which are not absorbed to any important extent. Thus when liquid paraffin is used as a laxative fat-soluble vitamins may be carried by it, in solution, into the faeces, and thus excreted.

VITAMINS OF THE B COMPLEX

Introduction

The original vitamin B, which was shown to cure the disease beri-beri, was later found to be associated in foods with another factor effective in curing pellagra. The anti-beriberi factor was called vitamin B_1, and the anti-pellagra factor vitamin B_2. Later, vitamin B_2 itself was shown to contain the anti-pellagra vitamin nicotinic acid, and riboflavin. Other dietary factors have since been assigned to the B group, among which are vitamin B_{12}, folic acid and vitamin B_6 or pyridoxine.

Function :- Metabolism of Carbohydrates + Release of energy from Carbohydrate esp for nerve cells

THIAMIN (vitamin B_1)

Functions

Thiamin constitutes part of an enzyme system concerned in the metabolism of carbohydrate. It is necessary for the metabolism of pyruvic acid, a substance which is produced during the breakdown of glycogen in the muscles to yield energy.

Dietary sources

Thiamin is found in many foods, but in small amounts. The best sources are the germinating parts of cereals and other plants. Wholemeal flour and bread are of importance for their thiamin content. Unfortified white flour, and bread made from such flour, contain relatively little thiamin, as it is removed with the germ and bran during milling of the wheat. In the United Kingdom, however, white flour is artificially fortified with the vitamin. Other moderately good sources are milk, eggs, liver, kidney, pork, peas and beans. Some proprietary breakfast cereals and cereal foods for infants are fortified with thiamin and yeast extracts are an excellent source.

Table 6.3 Vitamin B

Sources
Found especially in *fresh
unprocessed foods* and wholegrain
cereals

Functions
Thiamin, riboflavin and nicotinic
acid: components of *enzyme
systems* concerned in oxidation of
foodstuffs
....
Vitamin B$_{12}$ and folic acid: *red
blood cell* formation

Deficiency
Thiamin: *beriberi*
Riboflavin: *skin lesions corneal
vascularisation*
Nicotinic acid: *pellagra*
Vitamin B$_{12}$: pernicious *anaemia*
Folic acid: nutritional megaloblastic
anaemia

Effect of cooking

Thiamin is soluble in water and some loss occurs when cooking water is discarded. It is destroyed by alkalis and by very high temperatures. Ordinary cooking temperatures are not sufficiently high to cause much loss, but a considerable loss of thiamin occurs when bread is toasted.

Recommended intake

Thiamin is involved in carbohydrate metabolism so the requirement is related to the amount of carbohydrate in the diet.

The Committee on Medical Aspects of Food Policy advised, for average adults, intakes ranging from 0.7 to 1.3 mg daily. Details of these recommendations are given in Appendix 2.

Deficiency

Beri-beri

Lack of thiamin is believed to be the principal cause of the disease beri-beri, which occurs among people whose staple food is polished rice. The peripheral nerves are affected, resulting in a condition referred to as polyneuritis. The legs and feet particularly are involved and there is pain, weakness, degeneration of the muscles and inability to perform co-ordinated movements. This is known as dry beri-beri. In some cases fluid accumulates in the tissues (oedema) and the resultant swelling obscures the wasting of muscle. Heart function may be impaired and death can occur from heart failure. This form of the disease is known as wet beri-beri. Infantile beri-beri with cardiovascular symptoms occurs in breastfed infants if the diet of the mother is grossly deficient in thiamin. If the vitamin is provided in time these changes are reversed and little permanent injury remains.

It is believed that although thiamin deficiency is the principal cause of beri-beri, a lack of other dietary factors, particularly other vitamins of the B complex, plays a part in bringing about the condition. Treatment involves providing a diet adequate in all essential nutrients, with supplements of the vitamins of the B group, emphasis being placed on thiamin.

In the past beri-beri has been the cause of much disease and death. It was particularly prevalent among men at sea for long periods of time, who were unable to obtain fresh foods. Beriberi still occurs in the East in countries where highly refined rice is the staple food and very little fresh food is eaten.

In western countries polyneuropathy of nutritional origin has been reported in cases of chronic alcoholism associated with grossly defective diet. It has also been known to occur as a result of persistent vomiting during pregnancy and in association with disorders of the intestinal tract affecting the absorption of food.

 ## RIBOFLAVIN (vitamin B₂)

Function

Riboflavin is a constituent of a number of enzymes concerned in oxidation and reduction processes in body tissues.

helps responsible for metabolism of Carbohydrates.

Dietary sources

Riboflavin is found in many foods. The most valuable dietary source is milk. 500 ml supply half of the recommended daily intake for an average person. Other valuable sources are egg yolk, liver, kidney and heart. Some proprietary breakfast cereals and cereal foods for infants are fortified with riboflavin. Meat, fish, vegetables and whole grain cereals contain small amounts. Yeast has a high riboflavin content.

Effects of cooking, storage and preservation

This vitamin is not much affected by cooking, drying, canning or freezing of foods. It is sensitive to light and much of the riboflavin in milk is destroyed after several hours' exposure to sunlight. The riboflavin content of foods is reduced by the addition of alkalis such as baking soda, but not to the same extent as occurs in the case of thiamin.

Recommended intake

The Committee on Medical Aspects of Food Policy advised daily intakes of 1.6 mg for the average man and 1.3 mg for the average woman. Further details are given in Appendix 2.

Deficiency

The effects of riboflavin deficiency are apparent in the skin, particularly that of the face; also in the eye. They include inflammation of the lips and tongue, a waxy skin eruption around the nose and lips, and cracks at the corners of the mouth. The cornea of the eye is infiltrated by small blood vessels, producing a bloodshot appearance, and the eyes are painful and sensitive to light. These affections are not found only in association with riboflavin deficiency but are known to accompany other disorders.

Deficiency of riboflavin is believed to be rare in the United Kingdom. It is found in some parts of the East and when it occurs is usually associated with deficiency of thiamin, nicotinic acid and other factors.

✳ NICOTINIC ACID (niacin)

Function   *concerned in release of energy from carbohydrates*

Nicotinic acid, like riboflavin, is a component of enzyme systems concerned in oxidation and reduction processes in body tissues.

Dietary sources

Whole grain cereals and wholemeal bread, meat, liver, kidney, fish and pulse vegetables are all natural sources of this vitamin. It appears, however, that not all of the nicotinic acid occurring in cereals can be absorbed by the body. In the preparation of refined flours nicotinic acid is progressively removed during milling. However, in the United Kingdom, flours other than wholemeal are artificially fortified with the vitamin in an available form, with the result that flour products are an important source of nicotinic acid. Some proprietary breakfast cereals and cereal foods for infants are fortified with this vitamin. Yeast has a high nicotinic acid content. The amino acid tryptophan can be converted to nicotinic acid in the body and is thus a precursor of the vitamin.

Recommended intake

This vitamin is available from two sources; nicotinic acid ingested as such, and also its precursor the amino acid tryptophan. For this reason the Panel on Recommended Intakes suggested that it should be measured in nicotinic acid equivalents. One mg nicotinic acid equivalent is defined as being equal to 1 mg of available nicotinic acid or 60 mg tryptophan. An intake of 18 mg equivalents daily has been recommended for average men and 15 mg equivalents for average women. See Appendix 2 for further details.

✳ Deficiency

Deficiency of nicotinic acid is usually accompanied by deficiency of several vitamins of the B group. Other dietary factors may be lacking also. In the initial stages there is loss of weight and appetite accompanied by general ill-health. Prolonged deficiency gives rise to a condition known as pellagra. Reddish-brown pigmented areas appear on the skin, especially on areas which are exposed, such as the neck, face and hands, They occur equally on both sides of the body, giving a symmetrical appearance. There is inflammation of the gastrointestinal tract, resulting in diarrhoea. Mental changes include irritability, anxiety and depression, progressing in severe cases to hallucinations and dementia. Dermatitis, diarrhoea and dementia have become known as the 3Ds of pellagra. Symptoms resulting from a deficiency of other factors such as thiamin and riboflavin also occur.

This condition responds to a balanced diet with supplements of the missing factors.

Pellagra is a disease of predominantly maize-eating peoples. Maize is not a good dietary source of nicotinic acid; it also has a low tryptophan content. Pellagra is still seen in some countries, including India, Central Asia and parts of Africa.

PYRIDOXINE (vitamin B_6)

Vitamin B_6 consists of a number of related substances, one of which is called pyridoxine. It is important in amino acid metabolism.

Human deficiency is very rare but has been known to occur in certain infants who appear to have an increased requirement for the vitamin.

VITAMIN B_{12} (cyanocobalamin)

Function

Vitamin B_{12} is essential for the normal development of red blood cells. It has been shown to be the anti-anaemia factor first isolated from liver extracts, and used for the treatment of pernicious anaemia.

Gastric juice contains a secretion, so far unidentified, which assists absorption of this vitamin.

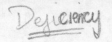 _Defuciency_

✳ Dietary sources

Liver, kidney and heart are particularly good sources of vitamin B_{12} and valuable amounts are present in muscle meats, fish, cheese and eggs. Milk contains a smaller, but useful amount. _green vegs._

Deficiency

A deficiency of vitamin B_{12} usually results from lack of the intrinsic factor necessary for its absorption. This may be seen in persons in whom gastric secretion is impaired, or who have had a complete gastrectomy. A condition suggestive of vitamin B_{12} deficiency is sometimes seen in strict vegetarians who eat no animal foods of any kind.

FOLIC ACID, (folate)

Function

Folic acid, like vitamin B_{12}, has been shown to be essential for the development of red blood cells, and is effective in the treatment of certain types of anaemia.

Dietary sources

It is widely distributed in foods in a variety of forms which are chemically related, and are known collectively as folate. Green leafy vegetables are a particularly rich source. It is not a stable vitamin and considerable losses occur during cooking.

Requirement

Requirement is increased during pregnancy. The megaloblastic anaemia which is sometimes observed in this condition, and which responds to treatment with folic acid, is due in part to defective diet. Folate deficiency sometimes occurs in premature babies, in association with the malabsorption syndrome, and in elderly persons living on poor diets. Dietary deficiency of folic acid giving rise to anaemia, occurs in tropical countries.

ASCORBIC ACID (vitamin C)

Functions

Ascorbic acid is required for the formation of the connective tissue, or intercellular material, in which the cells of the body are embedded. This vitamin also appears to be necessary for the formation of the red cells of the blood.

Dietary sources

Ascorbic acid is found principally in fresh fruits and vegetables. Good sources are oranges, grapefruit, lemons, tomatoes and leafy vegetables such as cabbage, broccoli, cauliflower and spinach. Blackcurrants, gooseberries, raspberries and strawberries contain considerable amounts of ascorbic acid, but their season is short. Other fruits contain small amounts. Potatoes and turnips have a comparatively small ascorbic acid content, but as they are staple foods they constitute a very important dietary source, especially for people who cannot afford the more expensive foods, or who through ignorance or neglect are living on a diet lacking in variety and containing insufficient of the vitamin from other foods. Milk has a low ascorbic acid content and this is still further reduced by pasteurisation. Rose hips are particularly rich in ascorbic acid and are used in the preparation of rose hip syrup, a concentrate sometimes used when a supplement of this vitamin is required.

Conservation of ascorbic acid in foods

Storage, preparation and cooking of foods can result in much loss of ascorbic acid, as this vitamin is soluble in water and also easily oxidised, especially in the presence of alkalis, and when exposed to heat or light.

The ascorbic acid content of foods is much reduced during storage. Thus new potatoes have a higher content of ascorbic acid than old ones which have been stored during the winter. Loss of ascorbic acid occurs when wilting takes place. Many fruits and vegetables contain an enzyme, ascorbic acid oxidase, which increases the rate of oxidation of ascorbic acid. This enzyme is brought into contact with the vitamin by

Table 6.4 Vitamin C

Sources
Certain *vegetables* and *fruits*

Functions
Necessary for formation of
connective tissue

Deficiency
Scurvy

bruising, shredding and grating. To ensure the maximum retention of the vitamin during the preparation of food for the table knowledge of these facts must be put to practical account. This aspect of the subject is dealt with more fully in Chapter 11.

Recommended intake

The Committee on Medical Aspects of Food Policy expressed the opinion that 30 mg ascorbic acid daily provide an adequate intake for average adult persons. This should be increased to 60 mg during pregnancy and lactation. Further details are given in Appendix 2.

Deficiency

In the initial stages deficiency of ascorbic acid gives rise to weakness, irritability, decreased resistance to infection and pains in the limbs and joints. Prolonged deficiency results in scurvy. This condition is characterised by multiple haemorrhages. It is usually accompanied by swollen, bleeding and inflamed gums. The gums, however, remain unaffected if no teeth are present. Spontaneous haemorrhages occur under the skin and are apparent as small red dots or patches, or as extensive areas of bruising. Haemorrhages also occur into the joints, under periosteal membranes and into the muscles. Degenerative changes take place in the bones. Anaemia is frequently present.

In infancy scurvy is characterised by painful, swollen joints. The limbs are tender and the child cries when being handled. Bone degeneration may give rise to deformities resembling those seen in rickets. Spontaneous haemorrhages may also occur.

Scurvy responds readily to a diet high in nutritive value, with additional ascorbic acid.

Incidence. Scurvy is known to have been the cause of disease and death for some hundreds of years. It has been of frequent occurrence in the United Kingdom and other North European countries. Early navigators, at sea for long periods of time, lost large numbers of men through death from scurvy. Armies have suffered its effects—Florence Nightingale reported a high incidence among the British troops during the war in the Crimea.

Today scurvy is no longer encountered on this scale, but may be seen occasionally in persons eating very restricted diets, for example old people living alone and unable to cater adequately for themselves. Infants, especially if artificially fed, are liable to develop scurvy if they are not given supplements of ascorbic acid, particularly if the introduction of mixed feeding is delayed. In the United Kingdom a supplement is available through the Welfare Foods Service. Varying degrees of ascorbic acid deficiency have been observed in the past in people on badly planned gastric diets, lacking in fruits and vegetables.

An increased need for this vitamin occurs when healing is taking place. Persons suffering from such disorders as peptic ulcer, or ulceration of the colon, or who have suffered burns, fractures, extensive operation or other injury, should be ensured an adequate intake, otherwise recovery will be delayed.

QUESTIONS

1. Which nutritional deficiences are most likely to occur in this country?
2. Which foods should be included in the diet to prevent them from developing?
3. Why is vitamin C important and which foods contain it?
4. Which foods contain B vitamins?
5. What is xerophthalmia and why does it occur?

7

Energy

SUMMARY

Protein, fat, carbohydrate and alcohol are all dietary energy sources.

The energy content of a food can be calculated from its composition: 1 g fat supplies approximately 37 kJ, 1 g alcohol—29 kJ, 1 g protein—17 kJ and 1 g carbohyrate—16 kJ

An individual's energy requirement depends on both his basal metabolic rate (BMR) and his activity. The BMR is influenced by age, sex, environmental temperature, disease and body composition. Any excess energy not needed for metabolism is converted to fat and stored in the adipose tissues.

Energy may be defined as the capacity to perform work.

It is manifested in various ways such as heat, electicity, light or mechanical energy.

It is never destroyed, but one form of energy may be converted to another. For example the energy of a waterfall may be converted to a current of electricity, which in its turn may appear as light or heat, or may be used to drive a machine.

ENERGY REQUIREMENT

Energy is required for the following processes:

1. Growth and maintenance of body tissues. The body requires energy for the activity which takes place in cells when tissues are formed from simpler components.

2. Maintenance of body temperature.

3. Involuntary muscle movement. Such movements as the heart beat, movements of the gastrointestinal tract and the movements of the muscle involved in respiration all require the expenditure of energy.

4. Voluntary muscle movement. Energy is needed for all voluntary activity such as the performance of work, walking and playing sport.

Sources of energy

Energy is obtained from the oxidation of the carbohydrates, fats and proteins of the diet, the traditional unit of measurement being the calorie. The amount of energy resulting from the oxidation of carbohydrates, fats and proteins can be measured in the laboratory and as a result of experiment we know that in the body:

1 g carbohydrate supplies 16 kJ (4 kcal) approximately.

1 g fat supplies 37 kJ (9 kcal) approximately.

1 g protein supplies 17 kJ (4 kcal) approximately.

1 g alcohol supplies 29kJ (7 kcal) approximately.

The amount of carbohydrate, fat and protein used for energy production at a given time depends upon the rate at which tissue activity or metabolism is taking place, and a convenient way of measuring metabolism is to measure the energy produced as a result of the oxidation of food.

Units of energy

One calorie is the amount of heat required to raise 1 g water through 1°C. The unit with which we are familiar is in fact the kilocalorie (kcal), usually referred to as a calorie for the sake of convenience.

In the International System of Units agreed in 1960, to which the United Kingdom subscribed, the calorie has been replaced by the joule. This is a unit of energy irrespective of the form in which it appears. For example it can denote heat, electrical energy, or mechanical energy. One calorie is equivalent to 4.184 joules (4.2.).

When considering comparatively small amounts of energy, as in average portions of individual foods, the kilojoule (kJ) is convenient. For larger amounts of energy, for example total daily requirement, the megajoule (MJ) which is equivalent to 1000 kJ is to be preferred.

Measurement of energy

The measurement of heat is known as calorimetry, and the energy production of an individual may be measured in either of two ways—direct calorimetry or indirect calorimetry.

Direct calorimetry. The person concerned is put into a specially insulated room where the heat given off by the body is collected by pipes of circulating water and is then measured. Any mechanical work performed is also measured, expressed in terms of joules and added to the heat production to give the total energy expenditure. This method is very accurate, and is suitable for lengthy experiments, but the apparatus is expensive and elaborate.

Indirect calorimetry is a simpler method based on the fact that carbon dioxide is produced when food is oxidised. In this case the amount of oxygen taken in and the amount of carbon dioxide breathed out in a given time are measured, and from this it is possible to calculate the amount of food which has been oxidised and the amount of energy produced.

Basal metabolism

Basal metabolism may be defined as the amount of energy required to carry out the basic processes of life such as cellular activity, heart beat and respiration. *at rest*.

Measurement of basal metabolic rate (BMR)

This is measured by a form of indirect calorimetry when the person is completely at rest, comfortably warm and in a post-absorptive state with digestive and metabolic activity reduced

1 gramme of fat produces 9.3 calories
" " " Carbohydrate " 4.1
" " " Protein " — 4.1

to a minimum. The BMR is related to lean body mass: for an average 65 kg man it is 4.8 KJ (1.14 kcal) per minute and for an average 55 kg woman 3.8 kJ (0.91 kcal) per minute approximately. Variation in the BMR occurs in certain pathologic conditions and BMR determinations are sometimes of value in the diagnosis of disease.

Total energy requirement

In order to carry out the activities of everyday life such as walking, going up and down stairs, doing housework, working in industry, or any form of activity, further energy is required in addition to that needed for basal metabolism. The total energy requirement for many activities has been measured by indirect calorimetry. A broad classification is given in Table 7.1. Such a classification is of course far from precise: for example the amount of energy expended rowing, playing football, or gardening will vary greatly depending upon the circumstances.

An experienced observer might assess the energy requirement of an average moderately active woman as follows:

In bed 8 hours (480 min)
  basal metabolism $480 \times 3.8 = 1824$ kJ (430 kcal)

Very light effort 12 hours
  (720 min) 6.3 kJ per min. $720 \times 6.3 = 4\,536$ kJ (1080 kcal)

Light effort 3½ hours (210 min)
  10.5 kJ per min. $210 \times 10.5 = 2205$ kJ (520 kcal)

Moderate effort ½ hour (30 min)
  25.2 kJ per min. $30 \times 25.2 = 756$ kJ (180 kcal)

_____

Total 9321 kJ (2220 kcal)
(9.3 MJ)

The energy recommendations of the Committee on Medical Aspects of Food Policy are reproduced in Appendix 2. These estimates are intended as a guide to those catering for large numbers of people and should not be applied rigidly to the needs of individuals. There are wide variations in energy needs even among those engaged in similar activities, and considerable deviations from these estimations are consistent with good health. The energy intake required for the main-

1,200 – 1,400 Kcal. – Women
1,600 – 1,800 Kcal – Men

Table 7.1 Approximate energy expenditure per minute, related to work

Very light less than 10 kJ (2.4 kcal)	Light 10–20 kJ (2.4–4.8 kcal)	Moderate 20–30 kJ (4.8–7.1 kcal)	Heavy 30–40 kJ (7.1–9.5 kcal)	Very heavy 40–50 kJ (9.5–11.9 kcal)
for example: floor sweeping preparing vegetables typing driving a lorry	for example: bed making window cleaning shopping with a light load welding washing up in a canteen	for example: cycling dancing gardening cabinet making shopping with a heavy load drilling coal or rock	for example: digging with pick and shovel cleaving wood rowing football	for example: boxing working with an axe, 35 blows per minute

tenance of a normal weight in the individual concerned is the best guide as to requirement.

Factors affecting energy requirement

We have already seen that basal requirement is affected by the size of the individual, that it is greater in men than in women, and that the total energy requirment depends upon the degree of muscular activity which is taking place. Various other factors remain to be considered.

1. Age. In children the BMR is higher per unit of surface area than in adults. BMR is lower in old age.

2. Enviromental temperature. Metabolism is increased in cold climates , resulting in increased heat production which helps to maintain body temperature.

3. Disease. In fevers the metabolic rate in increased by eight per cent approximately for every 0.5°C rise in temperature. Certain endocrine disorders affect BMR , for example, hyperthyroidism raises it and hypothyroidism lowers it.

4. Pregnancy. BMR is increased during pregnancy and lactation.

5. Energy intake. In prolonged undernutrition, the body compensates for the inadequate energy intake by a reduction in the metabolic rate.

Specific dynamic action of food

Food has the effect of stimulating the metabolic rate while it is being metabolised, thus causing increased energy expenditure. This is known as the specific dynamic action of food and varies with the type of food eaten. In a mixed diet it amounts to an increased expenditure of energy equal to about 10 per cent of the basal requirement. When accurate determination of energy requirement is being carried out this must be taken into consideration.

Effect of excess energy intake

If the diet eaten by an individual supplies more energy than required the excess food is used to make fat, which can be stored in the body in large amounts. This is the basic mechanism of obesity.

Energy value of a diet

By using tables giving the protein, carbohydrate and fat content of foods the composition and energy value of a diet can be calculated.

Example. Estimation of the approximate protein, fat and carbohydrate content, and total energy value, of one day's food intake.

Subject: A housewife

Menu

Breakfast
Cereal with milk.
Toast with butter and marmalade.
Coffee.

Mid-morning
Coffee.

Snack Lunch
Vegetable soup.
Bread roll as cheese and tomato sandwich.
Fresh Fruit.
Coffee with biscuits.

Mid-afternoon
Tea.
Scone with butter.

Evening meal
Stewed beef.
Turnip boiled
Potato boiled.
Apple Crumble and custard.
Tea.

Table 7.2

Total food Intake	Analysis For the purpose of this calculation weights of food portions are given to the nearest 5 g, and values for protein, fat and carbohydrate to the nearest whole number (Appendix 4)		
	Protein g	Fat g	Carbohydrate g
Cornflakes 20 g	2	neg.	17
Bread 120 g (3 rounds bread and 1 roll)	10	2	55
Scone 45 g (1 large)	3	7	25
Biscuits 30 g (1 Digestive and 2 Rich Tea)	2	5	22
Apple Crumble 90 g (2 tablesp.)	2	6	33
Custard 120 g (6 tablesp.)	4	5	20
Milk 380 ml (⅔pt)	12	14	18
Cheese 35 g	9	12	neg.
Beef stew 120 g	11	9	4
Vegetable soup 210 g (⅓pt)	3	1	14
Potato boiled 180 g (1 medium)	2	neg.	35
Turnip boiled 70 g (1 serving)	neg.	neg.	2
Tomato 60 g (1 medium)	1	neg.	2
Orange 125 g	1	neg.	11
Marmalade 25 g (2 teasp.)	neg.	0	17
Sugar 30 g	neg.	0	31
Butter 40 g	neg.	33	neg.
Totals	62	94	306

Total energy value—$(62 \times 17) + (94 \times 37) + (306 \times 16)$kJ or $1054 + 3478 + 4896 = 9.4$ MJ (2300 kcal approx.)

QUESTIONS

1. What is energy needed for?
2. Name three high energy foods.
3. List some factors which influence energy requirement.

8

Dietary fibre

SUMMARY

1. Dietary fibre is found in plants and cannot be digested by man.
2. It has many effects on the physiology of the gastrointestinal tract.
3. The Western diet has a low fibre content. This has been linked with an increased incidence of certain degenerative diseases.
4. Most people need to increase their daily fibre intake. It should come from wholemeal bread, wholegrain cereals, vegetables and fruit.

INTRODUCTION

'Soon none but the poor and ignorant will use white bread, brown bread is not a luxury but a necessity for every family'. This statement was published in a pamphlet which was widely circulated by Thomas Allinson. It was part of his campaign to persuade the Victorians to adopt a healthier way of life. His campaign was successful in some circles. In 1847, Queen Victoria responded to it by changing to wholemeal bread and encouraged her Court to do the same. In spite of this auspicious start the presence of fibre in foods and the importance of fibre in the diet was ignored for the next century. During that period the terms roughage and fibre were assumed to be synonymous. Fibre was considered to be usefully included in the diet only as a treatment for constipation. The ideal diet was supposed to be one which contained highly refined foods and was completely digested. It was only the robust whose digestive tract could survive the onslaught of roughage!

In the last 20 years clinical scientists have shown that fibre is an essential component of a well-balanced diet. It has many functions and not all of them are completely understood.

Definition of dietary fibre

Dietary fibre is that plant material which cannot be digested by the enzymes of the human gastrointestinal tract.

A wide variety of fibres are found in the plant kingdom. Fibres of many different types and in differing amounts are found in all plant structures. They are in the cell walls and within the cells of roots, leaves, stems, seeds and fruits.

Chemical composition of dietary fibre

Modern methods for the chemical analysis of dietary fibre show that it can be divided into three main groups.

1. Cellulose is a glucose polysaccharide which is the most common type of dietary fibre; the long tough fibrous strands give plants their form and rigidity and get stuck between man's teeth! Leafy vegetables are a rich source of cellulose.

2. Pectin, plant gums and mucilages have a similar composition. They are all non-cellulosic polysaccharides but have different functions in plants.

> *Pectins*—combine with water to form a gel. It is their presence in fruit that enables them to hold so much water, e.g. an orange is 85 per cent water.
>
> *Plant gums*—are produced by plants to cover and protect the site of an injury, e.g. the gum on a fir tree.
>
> *Mucilages*—are found mixed with the endosperm in the seeds of some plants. The mucilages are able to hold water which prevents seeds from drying out while

dormant. The seeds of peas and beans are rich sources of the mucilaginous fibres.

3. *Lignin* is the fibre that gives wood its characteristic form, structure and strength. The amounts of lignin in a tree varies between 10 to 50 per cent, the amount depends on the species and maturity of the tree. It is unimportant in the human diet.

Analysis of fibre in food

The fibre removed from cereals during milling has been used as animal feed for hundreds of years. The first method of analysis of dietary fibre was used to check that sawdust had not been added to animal feed. The value for dietary fibre content obtained by the old chemical analytical methods is called the *crude fibre content*. This term is used because it is now known that during analysis, a lot of pectin, gums and mucilages and some of the cellulose was destroyed leaving mainly the lignin to be measured. This explains why recent food tables show the dietary fibre content of the Western diet to be three times the previously measured (crude fibre) value.

Roughage is an old fashioned term which does not describe fibre adequately and should not be used. It suggests that fibre is an inert substance whose only function is to provide the gastrointestinal tract with a harsh, scratchy, bulking agent. This is not so. Dietary fibre is a complex mixture of substances which have a wide range of effects on the gastrointestinal tract.

EFFECTS OF DIETARY FIBRE ON THE GASTROINTESTINAL TRACT (See Fig. 8.1)

Mouth. Unrefined fibre-rich foods are coarse and bulky so they need to be chewed for longer than refined foods. The extra chewing stimulates increased salivation. Both the increased chewing and salivation help to keep the teeth and gums healthy.

Stomach. In general, unrefined fibre-rich foods stay in the stomach for longer than the refined form of the same food. This slowing of gastric emptying means that people feel fuller

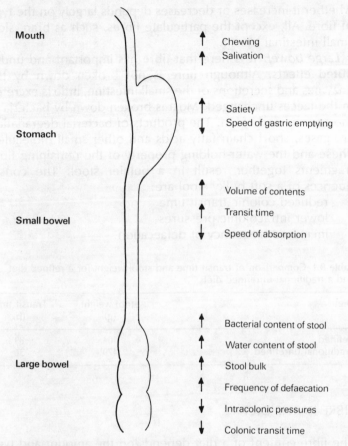

Mouth

↑ Chewing
↑ Salivation

↑ Satiety
↓ Speed of gastric emptying

Stomach

↑ Volume of contents
↑ Transit time
↓ Speed of absorption

Small bowel

↑ Bacterial content of stool
↑ Water content of stool
↑ Stool bulk
↑ Frequency of defaecation
↓ Intracolonic pressures
↓ Colonic transit time

Large bowel

Figure 8.1 Summary of the effects of dietary fibre on the gastrointestinal tract.

after a meal and so eat slightly less. It also means that food enters the small bowel more slowly, so digestion and absorption by the small bowel is slowed down.

Small bowel. Different types of fibre have different effects on the function of the small bowel. The group of fibres whose actions are best understood are the pectins, gums and mucilages. They increase the viscosity of the small bowel contents and slow the rate of absorption of the products of digestion. Though absorption is complete, it continues further down the small intestine than when fibre is absent.

Small bowel transit time is altered by most fibres, though

whether it increases or decreases depends largely on the type of fibre. All, except the particulate fibres, such as bran, slow small intestinal transit.

Large bowel. It is here that fibre has important and undisputed effects. Although fibre is not broken down by the enzymes and secretions of the small intestine, little is excreted in the faeces unchanged. Most is broken down by bacteria in the caecum and colon. The products of bacterial degradation are gases, short chain fatty acids and other small molecules. These and the water-holding property of the remaining fibre fragments together result in a bulkier stool. The consequences of a soft bulky stool are:

reduced colonic transit time
lower intracolonic pressures
increased frequency of defaecation.

Table 8.1 Comparison of transit time and stool weight for a refined diet and a traditional unrefined diet

Diet	Stool weight (g)	Transit time (h)
Refined	104	83
Traditional unrefined	470	36

FIBRE IN THE DIET

The fibre content of a diet depends on the amount and type of plant material eaten. In Figure 8.2, the bar charts compare the total intake of fibre and the sources of fibre in the diets of three different populations.

Although the average intake of dietary fibre in the United Kingdom is 20 g there is a wide variation. Vegetarians who have a high intake of fruit and vegetables, and usually eat whole grain cereals, have an average intake of 30 g a day. The type of dietary fibre as well as the amount eaten changes with changes in the agriculture and affluence of the population. In the United Kingdom the amount of cereal fibre in the diet has halved in the last 100 years. This has not been accompanied by a halving in total dietary fibre intake, as more fruit and

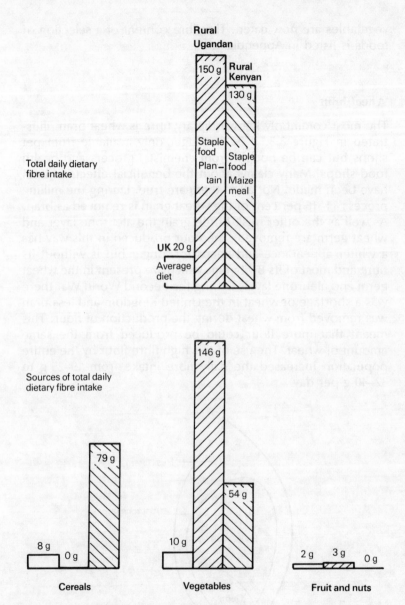

Figure 8.2 Comparison of fibre source and intake in the diets of three different populations.

vegetables are now eaten. The fibre content of a selection of foods is listed in Appendix 4.

Wheat bran

The most commonly known dietary fibre is wheat bran, illustrated in Figure 8.3. It is no longer only available from pet shops but can be bought from chemists, grocers and health food shops. Many claims about the beneficial effects of bran have been made. Not all of them are true. During the milling process 11–16 per cent of the wheat grain is removed as bran. As well as the outer husk of the grain the aleurone layer and wheat germ are removed. The flour produced in this way has a whiter appearance and keeps for longer but is without its fibre and most of its B vitamins which are present in the wheat germ and aleurone layer. During the Second World War there was a shortage of wheat in the United Kingdom and less bran was removed from wheat during the production of flour. This meant that more flour could be produced from the same amount of wheat. The use of this high fibre flour by the entire population increased the daily fibre intake from 19–25 g to 32–40 g per day.

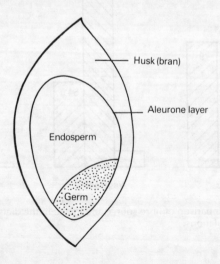

Figure 8.3 Wheat grain.

The fibre hypothesis

This was formulated in the 1970s by Burkitt and Trowell. Both of these men were doctors who had been working in East Africa for over 20 years. They observed that many of the degenerative diseases which were common in the United Kingdom were rare in Africa. They also noted that the rural Africans passed frequent bulky stools. In their hypothesis they related both of these observations to the type of diet eaten by the rural Africans and proposed 'that dietary fibre protects against a wide range of diseases'. The diseases which they suggested on epidemiological evidence were related to a low dietary fibre intake are listed below. The list is divided into three groups:

1. Colonic disorders
2. Disorders which are secondary to colonic disorders
3. Metabolic disorders.

Colonic disorders	Secondary disorders	Metabolic disorders
Constipation	Hiatus hernia	Obesity
Diverticular disease	Deep venous thrombosis	Diabetes
Colonic cancer	Pulmonary embolism	Atherosclerosis
Appendicitis		Gallstones

As these diseases are chronic and slow to develop, it is impossible to prove that their development is due to a fibre-deficient diet alone. Epidemiological studies have shown that in areas where there is a high intake of dietary fibre, the incidence of some of these diseases is low. However, it must be remembered that there are a multitude of differences between the life-styles of a rural African and a Western business man and that dietary fibre intake is only one of these. The considerable differences between the traditional diet of the rural African and that eaten in a developed country are summarised in Figure 8.4.

DIETARY FIBRE AND DISEASE

Colonic disorders

Constipation. No-one disputes the necessity of an adequate intake of dietary fibre for normal colonic function and the

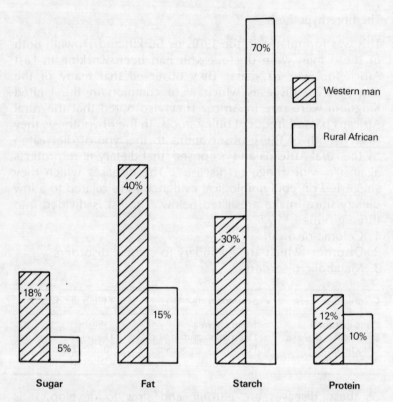

Figure 8.4 Percentages of total energy provided by sugar, fat, starch and protein: a comparison of two diets.

prevention of constipation. The effectiveness of different foods in increasing faecal weight and bulk depends on the type and amount of fibre they contain. For example, 50 g of wheat bran which contains 44 per cent fibre and 8 per cent water will double faecal weight, whilst 1500 g of eating apples which contain 2 per cent fibre and 84 per cent water are needed to have the same effect. The use of wheat bran for the treatment of constipation is discussed in Chapter 20, Diet in disorders of the gastrointestinal tract.

Diverticular disease. It has been suggested that diverticula form as a result of the high intracolonic pressures which occur in response to the constipation caused by diets low in fibre. Diets with a high-fibre content are used successfully to treat diverticular disease; the increased faecal volume and softer stool consistency lowers intracolonic pressures giving symptomatic relief and reducing the frequency of episodes of diverticular inflammation (diverticulitis). Lower intracolonic pressures also probably reduce the tendency to form more diverticula.

Colonic cancer. Epidemiological evidence links the intake of dietary fibre with the incidence of colonic cancer. It has been suggested that a fibre-rich diet may be protective against colonic cancer. The proposed mechanisms are:

1. Fibre binds potential carcinogens and removes them from the colon
2. The increased faecal bulk dilutes the concentration of carcinogens present
3. The reduced transit time reduces the length of time that the colon is exposed to carcinogens.

Secondary disorders

Hiatus hernia, haemorrhoids and varicose veins. The high intra-abdominal pressures which develop during straining to evacuate constipated stools may contribute to the development of these disorders. A high-fibre diet resulting in softer stools reduces straining and thus problems associated with these conditions. These disorders may also develop less commonly in those on a high-fibre diet.

Metabolic disorders

Obesity. During the last 40 years the amount of body fat in the adult population of the United Kingdom has increased by 10 per cent. Many changes in life-style have occurred all of which contribute to this increase. The increased consumption of fat and sugar is a more important cause of obesity than the decrease in fibre consumption. Many claims have been made about the value of dietary fibre as an aid to weight reduction. The addition of extra fibre to the diet increases the amount of energy, or dietary calories, excreted in the faeces. This loss is only slight and of negligible value to slimmers. The inclusion of unrefined high fibre foods in a calorie-controlled diet has two advantages: (1) they are tough and bulky so they take longer to eat; and (2) as the food stays in the stomach longer

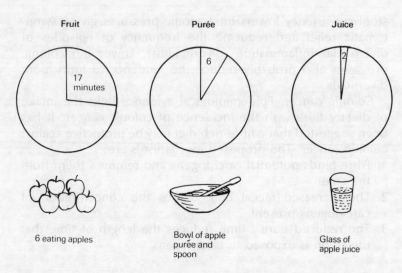

Figure 8.5 The times taken to eat six apples in three different forms.

it prolongs the feeling of fullness after a meal. Figure 8.5 shows the different times taken to eat apples in three different forms.

Diabetes mellitus. In regions where the diet is based on fibre-rich starchy foods the incidence of this disease is low. When people migrate from these regions to areas where the diet is rich in refined sugary foods, the incidence of diabetes increases, particularly the non-insulin dependent type (Type 2), along with the incidence of obesity and dental caries. The effect of fibre on slowing absorption has already been mentioned. The fibres which have the greatest influence on carbohydrate absorption are the viscous fibres. These occur naturally in legumes. Diets containing large amounts of legumes and diets containing the viscous fibre guar gum have been used to treat diabetes by slowing carbohydrate absorption, with varying degrees of success.

Heart disease. The link between heart disease and fibre intake is still unclear. The addition of some types of fibre, but not all types, will alter lipid metabolism and there is a low incidence of coronary heart disease amongst rural African populations.

Gall stones. Some fibres bind bile acids. This means that the bile acids are excreted with the fibre in the stool instead of being reabsorbed and recirculated in the enterohepatic circulation. By preventing the bile from becoming supersaturated this may prevent the formation of gall stones.

The disadvantage of fibre in the diet

Mineral deficiencies. The minerals calcium, magnesium, zinc, phosphorus and iron in the diet become partly bound to dietary fibre. Since the diet normally contains these minerals in excess, the body is able to adapt, by absorbing more. Deficiency of these minerals will only occur if the dietary intake is limited and nutritional status and body stores are already poor. For example, the addition of bran to the diets of some elderly people may precipitate osteomalacia in those with a low calcium and vitamin D intake, particularly if they are housebound.

Wind. Most people experience the symptoms of abdominal distention, discomfort and wind after increasing their intake of dietary fibre. This is due to the production of gas in the caecum and colon. Bacterial enzymes metabolise the fibre in the caecum and colon and produce the gases methane, hydrogen and carbon dioxide. The amount of gas produced depends on the type of fibre eaten and the bacterial flora present. The fibres and unabsorbable sugars found in peas and beans, for example, cause more wind than the fibre in bran. The large bowel and its bacteria gradually adapt to the high-fibre intake and the problem of wind usually lessens but never disappears.

QUESTIONS

1. Why do some people on a weight-reducing diet find high-fibre foods useful?
2. How does dietary fibre prevent constipation?
3. What is bran?
4. A meal containing dried peas and beans cause flatulence. Why?

9

Diet-related disease

SUMMARY

The treatment of disease by changing the patient's diet is not the only way in which diet and disease are linked. Diets which are nutritionally inadequate lead to the development of well-recognised deficiency diseases. Epidemiological evidence associates diet with an increased incidence of cardiovascular disease and cancer of the stomach, colon, breast and ovary. The dietary factor most frequently associated with increased disease incidence is total fat content.

INTRODUCTION

The association of diets deficient in essential nutrients with specific dietary deficiency diseases and of the use of diet as the treatment for certain diseases are both accepted and well established. However, the role of diet in causing or contributing to the cause of disease is less well understood. This relationship is important in the aetiology of many of the non-infectious diseases which are the major causes of death and ill health in the Western World.

Diets and disease are related in three ways:
1. The use of diet as a treatment for disease
2. Diseases which are caused by diet
3. Diseases whose incidence is associated with diet.

1. The use of diet as a treatment for disease

Special dietary modifications are used to treat a range of diseases. These diets do not usually cure the disease, they are used to correct metabolic abnormalities and to prevent or at least reduce symptoms. For example, the carefully controlled carbohydrate intake of the diabetic diet provides carbohydrate in amounts which can be metabolised using the available insulin, and the use of gluten-free foods in gluten sensitive enteropathy (coeliac disease) excludes the toxic agent gluten from the diet. There are many other ways in which diet is used to treat disease; they are explained in detail in later chapters.

2. Diseases which are caused by diet

Diet can cause disease when it contains too little or too much of a specific nutrient, if it contains dietary toxins, or when the food eaten is contaminated. One of the first diseases proved scientifically to be caused by diet was scurvy, which was common among sailors in the eighteenth century. James Lind was able to show that the addition of citrus fruits to the diet both cured and prevented scurvy. He also showed that other dietary and medicinal treatments were ineffective. Excessive intakes of nutrients which cannot be metabolised and excreted, such as the fat-soluble vitamins, also cause disease. These disorders along with the deficiency diseases are described in the chapters on specific nutrients.

The presence of poisonous substances in the diet can also cause disease. These can be naturally occurring substances in the food or formed in the food by processing, or they can be added to food unintentionally.

An example of naturally occurring toxins are the goitrogens which occur in cabbages and turnips and inhibit iodine absorption causing goitre of the thyroid gland. Legumes and some cereals also contain substances known as anti-nutrients which inhibit digestion and absorption of specific nutrients.These may cause malabsorption and its symptoms, but rarely cause clinical disease. Some foods contain chemicals which can be toxic when consumed in large amounts. In the processing of food, substances may be formed which are harmful, for example hydrocarbons formed during the smoking of foods and by high temperature frying. Chemical additives are frequently accused of causing disease though they rarely do. In the United Kingdom, the EEC, North America and most westernised countries, food processing is controlled by legislation and food additives are checked thoroughly for toxic effects before they are used.

In storage and preparation the diet can become contaminated with toxic substances such as bacteria, pesticides and heavy metals. Bacterial food poisoning is an acute disease which is easily identified. Other contaminants are less easily identified because the symptoms are less well known and take longer to develop.

3. Diseases whose incidence is associated with diet

The disease pattern of the Western world has changed considerably in the last 150 years. Better hygiene, improved living standards and treatment with antibiotics have reduced the incidence of infectious diseases. It is now necessary to identify the causes of the large group of degenerative diseases, such as diseases of the cardiovascular system, and various malignant diseases. The incidence of these diseases is increasing and has been linked to the diet of Western man. It is unlikely that these diseases are due to any one nutritional factor but rather to a combination of factors, some of which are nutritional. Most of the evidence to associate diet with disease is epidemiological.

EPIDEMIOLOGY

Early epidemiologists studied outbreaks of diseases such as cholera and typhoid. By studying these epidemics they were able to understand the disease better by identifying both the source of infection and the way in which it was spread.

Modern epidemiologists study the distribution of all disease, not only infectious ones, within a population and try to identify factors which influence them. These factors include geographical location, climate, age, income, occupation, ethnic group and diet. It is always difficult to identify one particular factor because many may be involved.

For example, the incidence of bowel disease amongst African bushmen is lower than amongst Western businessmen. This could be because the diet of businessmen is different, or because they drive to work, or even that they own a home computer, or any of a host of other factors. Epidemiological evidence can suggest causes which are associated statistically with a disease and may identify relationships between disease and environment but it rarely provides conclusive proof. Experimental evidence is needed to confirm a hypothesis. This is very difficult to obtain because the degenerative and malignant diseases take a long time to develop in man and evidence from animal experiments is not always directly applicable to man. Evidence from epidemiological studies does not necessarily mean that an individual exposed to a specific environmental factor will develop a disease. It indicates that the incidence of a disease among the population exposed to that factor is higher than the incidence in a population not exposed. Increased incidences of both cardiovascular disease and some malignant diseases have been associated with diet and are discussed below.

Diet and cardiovascular disease

A common cause of death in the United Kingdom is coronary artery disease. Millions of working days are lost each year as a result of diseases of the heart and blood vessels. The increase has been so marked that it is often referred to as the twentieth century epidemic. However, not every middle aged man in the United Kingdom will suffer a heart attack. Factors have been identified which appear to increase the risk of cardiovascular disease. The most important of these risk factors are cigarette smoking, hypertension and raised serum cholesterol. The link between diet and raised serum cholesterol is well documented. The most important factor is a high dietary intake of animal fat which leads to raised serum lipids.

It is low density lipoprotein (LDL) cholesterol fraction which is associated with an increased risk of heart disease. The cholesterol content of the diet is only important if it is high or if an individual is especially susceptible to it.

Other dietary factors which have been linked to cardiovascular disease are low dietary fibre, high sugar, protein and salt content in the diet, soft drinking water and a high ratio of saturated to polyunsaturated fats.

The diets of populations with a low incidence of cardiovascular disease are generally lower in fat, sugar, animal protein and salt and contain more fibre. Dietary fibre may have a protective effect as some fibres have a blood lipid lowering effect. The development of hypertension in some individuals is linked to dietary salt intake.

Diet and malignant disease

It has been suggested that 70 per cent of all malignant diseases are due to environmental factors. Diet has been implicated in many of these. Cancers of the stomach, colon, breast and ovary have all been linked specifically to diet. Their incidence is not associated with a high intake of one specific food but to the overall balance of nutrient content of the diet.

Gastric cancer

The incidence of this disease correlates well with the nitrite content of the diet. Nitrites and nitrates are used to preserve food, particularly meat. They are converted in the stomach to nitrosamines which are known to be carcinogenic under some circumstances. The countries with the highest incidence of gastric cancer are Chile and Colombia where the water has a high nitrate content, and Japan, where the diet is rich in salted and smoked dried foods. Its incidence in England and Wales has declined in recent years though the reason why is not clear. It may be due to the change to refrigeration as a means of food preservation. A diet rich in fruit and vegetables is associated with a low incidence of this disease. Experiments have shown that ascorbic acid inhibits nitrosamine formation and this may be part of the explanation.

Large bowel cancer

The link between this and fibre intake is discussed in Chapter 8. Some populations which take a low fibre, high fat diet, certainly have an increased incidence of colonic cancer. However, the relationship is not a simple causative one. A high fat diet increases the production of bile acids and this increases the faecal bile acid content. These bile acids can be converted to substances which are known experimentally to be carcinogens. A high fibre diet may be protective against their action by decreasing transit time, binding bile salts and increasing stool bulk thus diluting their concentration.

Breast and ovarian cancers

Epidemiological evidence shows that both of these diseases are more common among women eating a Western type diet than in women eating an unrefined, low fat diet. Dietary fat does not act directly as a carcinogen but may act indirectly by altering hormonal balance and by contributing to the development of obesity. Both of these diseases are oestrogen dependent and are also associated with obesity which is known to cause an increase in oestrogen production.

QUESTIONS

1. List five diet-related diseases and explain how diet affects them.
2. Why is the fat content of the diet important in relation to causing disease?
3. Epidemiology does not prove a diet/disease relationship but suggests possible mechanisms. Why is this?

10

Nutritive value of foods commonly eaten; new sources of food

SUMMARY

Diets contain a wide variety of foods. Different foods contain different nutrients in different amounts. It is important to know the nutritional content of foods so that any deficiencies can be anticipated and corrected.

In this section foods which are commonly eaten are considered, with reference to their most important constituents.

CEREALS *4 portions*

Cereals, such as wheat, oats, rice, barley and maize, are important sources of:

Carbohydrate in the form of starch.

Dietary fibre—bran.

Minerals especially iron and phosphorus.

Vitamins of the B complex especially thiamin and nicotinic acid.

Protein. This is present in a relatively small amount when compared with high protein foods such as meat. However, because of the quantity eaten, bread and other cereal products make an important contribution to our intake of protein.

These nutrients are not uniformly distributed throughout the grain, and the nutritive value of the cereal depends upon the degree of refinement which has taken place during milling.

Flour and bread

Extraction rate

The staple cereal food of Western people is wheat, which is converted to flour by milling. Extraction rate is the term used to indicate the proportion of the wheat grain which is retained in the flour.

In the case of flour made from the whole of the wheat grain the extraction rate is 100 per cent. In the preparation of flours of lower extraction rates varying amounts of the outer layers of the grain and the germ or embryo are excluded. These parts between them contain some of the most valuable nutrients in the grain, including most of the thiamin and iron (found principally in the germ), most of the nicotinic acid and phosphorus (mainly found in the outer layers) and protein of relatively high biological value. The outer layers also contain most of the bran, and a pigment which is responsible for the colour of higher extraction flours. The removal of this pigment results in the production of a whiter flour.

It will be seen, then, that the lower the extraction rate the whiter flour will be, but the less it will contain of certain important nutrients, notably thiamin, nicotinic acid and iron; also bran. The extraction rates for flours are:

white flour	60–70 per cent
brown flour	85–95 per cent
wholemeal flour	100 per cent

The term wheatmeal is sometimes used for brown flour.

Fortification of flour

Since the Second World War the nutritive value of flour has been to a certain extent safeguarded by legislation. The Bread and Flour Regulations, 1963, at present in force, provide that all flour sold for human consumption shall contain not less than certain specified minimum amounts of thiamin, nicotinic acid and iron. Thus the lower-extraction flours are fortified with these nutrients. The Regulations also provide for the addition of calcium to all flours other than those derived from the whole of the products of the milling of the wheat. When comparison is made between flours of varying extraction rates it must be remembered that the higher extraction flours contain more phytic acid than white flour, and that phytic acid combines with minerals such as iron and calcium to form insoluble salts which are not readily available to the body. On the other hand high extraction flours contain most of the bran, and are a better source of vitamins than white flour, even when the latter is fortified to the required level.

To summarise, it may be said that flour is of value chiefly as a source of:

1. starch
2. vitamins of the B complex, especially thiamin and nicotinic acid
3. iron
4. calcium, with the exception of 100 per cent extraction flour
5. protein
6. bran, especially brown and wholemeal flours.

Much of the iron, B vitamins and calcium are the result of fortification.

Bread is a valuable source of the various important nutrients present in flour and contributes 12 per cent of the energy content of the average United Kingdom diet. In the preparation of biscuits, scones, cakes and puddings the nutritive value is modified by the inclusion of ingredients such as eggs, fat, milk and fruit.

DAIRY PRODUCE

Milk

Milk for human consumption is obtained from a variety of animals, for example the cow, goat, reindeer, ewe and mare. Custom varies in different parts of the world, depending upon which animal is most readily available. All types of milk resemble one another in composition, but the constituents are present in varying proportions, depending upon the species from which the milk has been obtained. Thus cow's milk contains a higher proportion of protein than mare's milk. Cow's milk will be considered here as it is the most frequently used.

Milk is one of the most nutritious of foods. The most important constituents are:

1. *proteins*, principally casein and lactalbumin; milk proteins supply the essential amino acids in especially good proportions for tissue building
2. *carbohydrate*, in the form of lactose or milk sugar
3. *fat* in a finely emulsified form
4. *calcium and phosphorus*, in this case readily absorbed
5. *vitamin A*, in largest amount when the cow is eating green fodder high in carotene
6. *vitamins of the B complex*, especially riboflavin.

Although of high nutritive value milk is not a perfect food, as is sometimes supposed. Certain nutrients are poorly represented, notably iron, ascorbic acid and vitamin D.

Milk can be served in many different ways, requires the minimum of preparation, and is inexpensive when compared with other foods of comparable nutritive value. These considerations, along with the high biological value of its proteins, make it of particular value when a high protein diet is required.

One pint of milk contains the following nutrients:
   20 g protein
   22 g fat
   28 g carbohydrate
   700 mg calcium

Dried milk

Dried milk is prepared by passing the milk in a film between heated rollers or by spraying it through a fine nozzle into a heated drying chamber.

Dried milk, when reconstituted, is similar to fresh milk in nutritive value. There is some loss of thiamin and ascorbic acid. These losses, however, are not nutritionally significant.

Condensed and evaporated milks

In the preparation of condensed milk the milk is pasteurised, sugar is added and a proportion of the water content is removed by evaporation. Unsweetened condensed milk is also obtainable and is usually referred to as evaporated milk. The sweetened product owes its preservation to condensation and to the high sugar content, which inhibits bacterial growth. The preservation of the unsweetened condensed milk depends upon its having been sterilised after the sealing of the can.

Condensed milk, like the dried product, shows some loss of thiamin and ascorbic acid. These losses, however, do not significantly affect the nutritional value of the milk, as these vitamins are readily available from other sources.

Skimmed milk and cream

In the preparation of cream the fat is removed from milk either by a mechanical separator or by skimming by hand after the cream, or fat-containing portion has risen to the surface. The residue is known as skimmed milk or separated milk.

Cream has a high fat content and is of value principally as a source of energy. It is a suitable food for invalids as it is easily digested.

Skimmed milk is similar to whole milk in its content of carbohydrate, protein, minerals and water-soluble vitamins, but is of course lacking in fat and fat-soluble vitamins as these are removed with the cream. Because of its lower fat content, skimmed milk has a lower energy content than whole milk.

    1 pint skimmed milk   795 kJ (184 kcal)
    1 pint pasteurised whole milk   1523 mJ (364 kcal)

Some skimmed milk products are fortified with vitamins A and D.

Semi-skimmed milk

Only half of the fat has been removed in its preparation so the milk has a fat and energy content which is lower than whole milk but higher than skimmed milk.

Dried skimmed milk

When reconstituted this has a similar nutritional content to fresh skimmed milk. An exception to this is the dried skimmed milks with added vegetable fat. The fat added is not polyunsaturated. These milks have the advantage of being easy to reconstitute but are neither low in fat nor low in saturated fat.

Butter and buttermilk

In the preparation of butter, cream is subjected to continuous agitation known as churning. During this process the particles of fat come together to form butter.

Traditionally, butter was prepared from milk which had first been soured, the liquid remaining after removal of the fat being known as buttermilk. At the present time butter is prepared from fresh cream. Buttermilk available commercially has been made by adding to skim milk a culture of organisms which ferment lactose, resulting in lactic acid formation and imparting a characteristic sour flavour.

Butter has a high content of vitamin A, varying with the diet of the cow. The vitamin D content is moderate or low, being greater in summer than in winter.

Buttermilk is similar to skim milk in nutritive value.

Yoghurt

Yoghurt is made by adding to milk a specially prepared culture of bacteria which ferment the milk sugar lactose, giving rise to the production of lactic acid. Clotting takes place when a certain degree of acidity is reached. Flavour and food value are sometimes modified by the addition of such items as sugar, flavouring and fruit.

In general the food value of yoghurt is similar to that of milk, which is the basic constituent, but the information given on the container should be consulted in each case for detail of additional ingredients.

Cheese

In the preparation of cheese, milk is treated with rennet, an enzyme which brings about clotting. The clot is then broken up and separated into the liquid part, or whey, and the curd, which is solid. Cheese represents the curd, which has been salted, compressed and left for a period of time to ripen. During the ripening process chemical changes which take place modify the flavour of the cheese. In the preparation of most cheese the milk undergoes a preliminary ripening before the addition of the rennet. This is usually effected by adding a bacterial starter consisting of a culture of organisms which ferment lactose with the production of lactic acid. Cheeses are often named for their place of origin, examples being the well-known Cheddar and Cheshire varieties. A distinctive flavour can be imparted by encouraging the penetration of moulds, as is done in the case of Stilton, Danish Blue and Gorgonzola.

Most cheeses are excellent sources of protein, fat, calcium, phosphorus and vitamin A. Some riboflavin is also present. When cheese is prepared from skim milk the fat and vitamin A contents are much reduced. On the other hand cream cheese has a relatively high fat content.

Cottage cheese is prepared from skimmeo milk. Some fat is usually added to improve the texture. Fat content, however, s low, but will depend on the brand.

I cream

Ic cream is a frozen dessert consisting largely of milk or dried mi powder with the addition of sugar and often vegetable oil.The composition of the commercial product in respect of fat ontent and milk solids other than fat is controlled by legislatioı. When the fat of ice cream consists solely of butter fat, the poduct is referred to as Dairy Ice Cream.

Eggs

Eggs have a high nutritive value. They are of particular importance as a source of iron, and protein of high biological value, and contain considerable amounts of fat, calcium, phosphorus, vitamins A and D, thiamin and riboflavin. Most of these nutrients are present either wholly or principally in the yolk, the white contributing mainly protein and riboflavin. The protein of egg white is egg albumin, and the principal protein of the yolk is vitellin. Of all the dietary proteins, those found in eggs have the highest biological value. Egg yolk is a rich source of cholesterol, each yolk contains approximately 250 mg.

MARGARINE, COOKING FATS AND OILS

Margarine and cooking fat are prepared by the hydrogenation of vegetable oils, such as palm and maize oils (Chapter 3). Fish oils and other animal fats such as lard are also used. Not all margarines are low in cholesterol and high in polyunsaturated fat. Those margarines manufactured from a polyunsaturated vegetable oil are usually labelled 'high in polyunsaturates'.

The flavour of margarine is mainly determined by the addition of milk which has been cultured with selected organisms.

By law, margarine intended for the retail trade is fortified with vitamins A and D, and is in fact similar to butter in vitamin A content. It is a better source than butter of vitamin D. Cooking oils are blends of vegetable oils. Margarine, cooking fats, oils, and butter are similar in fat content and energy value. Low fat spreads contain less fat than margarine or butter and have a lower energy content.

MEAT   2 portions

The term meat usually implies beef, pork, mutton, veal or lamb. The greater part of meat is skeletal muscle, but the term may be extended to include offal. Poultry, game and rabbit may also be classified as meat.

The most important constituents of meat are protein, iron and B group vitamins, especially nicotinic acid. Varying amounts of fat are also present. Pork is a good source of thiamin.

Offal

Liver and brains have a high cholesterol content. Liver, kidney and heart have a comparatively high content of riboflavin, thiamin, nicotinic acid and iron. Liver especially is a good source of iron. It also has a high content of vitamin A.

The characteristic flavour and aroma of meat are due to the presence of organic substances known as extractives. These are of negligible nutritive value, but are important nevertheless as they stimulate the appetite and encourage the flow of digestive juices.

FISH   3 039

The flesh of fish is comparable with meat in composition. Like meat, it is a valuable source or protein and vitamins of the B group, especially nicotinic acid. Iron is also present, but to a much lesser extent than in meat.

In the case of dark-fleshed fish such as herrings, mackerel, sardines and salmon, fat is present between the muscle fibres. These are known as the fat, or oily fish, and supply not only fat, but valuable amounts of the fat-soluble vitamins A and D. The flesh of white fish such as cod, haddock, whiting, plaice and sole has a very low fat content, and contains a greater proportion of water than that of the dark-fleshed fish. It is therefore relatively lower in energy value. Some fish liver oils contain very high concentrations of vitamins A and D, e.g. cod and halibut liver oils.

The cooking of fish in fat, as in frying and grilling, adds greatly to its energy value.

VEGETABLES   4 portions

All vegetables have a structural framework of cellulose which is not digested and forms part of the faeces.

Unless artificially dried they have a high water content. The water content of green vegetables is around 90 per cent, of roots 80 to 90 per cent, of potatoes, peas and beans 70 to 80 per cent.

The vitamin content of vegetables is affected by cooking. This factor is dealt with in Chapter 12.

Green vegetables and tomatoes

Green vegetables contain varying amounts of vitamin C. Cabbage, cauliflower, broccoli, Brussels sprouts and tomatoes are important sources of this vitamin.

Tomatoes and vegetables with dark-green leaves, such as cabbage and spinach, are good sources of carotene, the precursor of vitamin A.

Green vegetables also contribute to the intake of iron and calcium.

The members of this group are of negligible energy value.

Potatoes

Potatoes when eaten in considerable amounts make a useful contribution to the energy value of the diet. One small potato, about 100 g in weight, is of approximately the same energy value as 30 g of bread or one thin slice—about 335 kJ (80 kcal).

The ascorbic acid content of potatoes is not great and decreases during storage. When regularly eaten, however, potatoes constitute an important source of this vitamin. They also contain small but significant amounts of protein, iron and B complex vitamins.

Root vegetables

Root vegetables such as carrot, turnip, parsnip and beetroot contain some ascorbic acid, but are not such a good source of this vitamin as the green vegetables. Turnips and swedes are the only really valuable sources of ascorbic acid in this group.

Carrots are of value as a source of carotene.

Root vegetables have a slightly higher energy value than greens, owing to the presence of a higher proportion of starch and sugar. Their contribution to the energy intake is nevertheless not very significant. Beetroot and parsnips contain more carbohydrate than carrots, turnips or swedes.

Pulse vegetables

Peas, beans and lentils contain more carbohydrate and protein than most other vegetables. Their protein, however, is of low biological value. They also contain considerable amounts of iron and B complex vitamins, especially thiamin. Fresh green peas and beans are a source of ascorbic acid.

FRUITS

Fruits contain varying amounts of ascorbic acid, but only some are good sources of this vitamin. Citrus fruits such as oranges and grapefruit have a high ascorbic acid content. Blackcurrants, strawberries, raspberries and gooseberries are also good sources, especially blackcurrants, but these fruits have a short season. The ascorbic acid content of blackcurrants is well retained, however, in the canned product, and in commercially prepared blackcurrant syrup.

Peaches, apricots and prunes are rich in carotene.

Some fruits have a high iron content, notably canned and dried peaches, dried apricots and figs, prunes, raisins, currants and sultanas. The extent to which this iron is available for absorption is, however, uncertain.

Fruits contain some carbohydrate, principally in the form of fructose.

As with vegetables, they have a structural framework of cellulose. The water content of the edible portion is usually high, e.g. approximately 94 per cent in the case of melon, 84 per cent in the case of apple and 86 per cent in the case of orange.

NUTS

Nuts, with the exception of the chestnut, have a high content of fat and protein and are moderately low in carbohydrate. They have therefore a high energy value. Other constituents include iron and B group vitamins. Chestnuts are comparatively low in fat and protein and high in carbohydrate.

Nuts are not eaten to any great extent in the United Kingdom, but are of great importance in vegetarian diets.

BEVERAGES

Tea and coffee are of no nutritive value apart from the addition of milk, cream or sugar. They contain caffeine, which is a mild stimulant, and not harmful in moderation. Taken in excess they sometimes cause sleeplessness and irritability.

Cocoa contains significant amounts of iron, protein, fat and carbohydrate, but in the amounts in which cocoa is normally consumed it is of little value as a source of these nutrients.

Meat extracts are stimulating to the appetite and encourage the flow of digestive secretions. They contain a considerable amount of certain of the vitamins of the B group. Their protein content is insignificant. They are used for flavouring soups and gravies, and also, diluted with water, as a beverage. Bovril is an example of a preparation which has a basis of meat extract.

Yeast extracts are similar in flavour to extracts of beef and have similar uses. They are good sources of the vitamins of the B group. An example of yeast extract is Marmite.

Alcoholic beverages

On metabolism, alcohol yields 29 kJ (7 kcal) per gram.

The alcohol content of beverages is variable, being approximately 5 per cent in the case of beer, cider and stout, around 10 per cent in the case of light wines and about 15 per cent in the case of sherry and port. Whisky, prepared by distilling a liquor resembling beer, and brandy, a distillate of wine, contain 30 to 40 per cent alcohol.

Sweet wines, beer and stout have a considerable carbohydrate content. Cider, ale, beer and stout have a high energy value, e.g., 500 ml stout provides approximately 840 kJ (200 kcal).

The regular, heavy and prolonged consumption of alcohol over a period of years can cause damage to certain organs, particularly the liver.

NEW SOURCES OF FOOD

One of the most serious problems facing us to-day is the feeding of a rapidly expanding world population, and one of

Table 10.1 Nutritive value of foods

Protein	Fat	Carbohydrate	Calcium	Iron	Vitamin A	Vitamin D	Thiamin	Riboflavin	Nicotinic acid	Ascorbic acid
Milk	Milk, butter and cheese	Flour: bread cakes	Milk	Eggs	Milk, butter and cheese	Oily fish	Widely distributed in foods, especially— flour and bread oatmeal bacon and pork peas and beans dried yeast	Milk	Flour and bread	Oranges
Cheese			Cheese	Liver		Fish Liver oils				Grapefruit
Eggs	Eggs	Porridge and other cereal foods	Flour and bread (except 100 per cent extraction)	Muscle meats	Eggs	Vitaminised margarine		Eggs	Meat and fish	Summer fruits: strawberries raspberries blackcurrants
Meat	Meat fat: dripping suet lard			Green vegetables	Vitaminised margarine			Yeast and yeast extracts		
Fish		Sugar: preserves confectionery	Hard water	Flour and bread	Oily fish	Butter			Yeast and meat extracts	Potatoes
Cereals						Eggs	Yeast extracts: Marmite	Meat extracts: Bovril		Turnips
Pulse vegetables	Margarine	Fruits			Fish liver oils					Swedes
Nuts	Cooking fat				Carotene: Carrots	Non-dietary source: Action on skin of ultra violet light				Tomatoes
	Baked products	Vegetables: potatoes dried peas and beans lentils beetroot parsnip			Tomatoes		Fortified cereals	Fortified cereals	Fortified cereals	Green vegetables
	Confectionery	Milk			Dark green leafy vegetables					Cauliflower

its most urgent aspects is the provision of sufficient protein in areas of greatest need. The situation is complicated by the fact that the production of protein in its most nutritious and acceptable forms, such as eggs, meat and milk, requires the feeding of crops to animals. This involves considerable wastage as the efficiency of conversion of plant protein to animal protein is only around 25 per cent.

The problem can be approached in numerous ways; for example by improvements in animal husbandry, reduction of wastage due to pests and other forms of spoilage, and by making fuller use of existing resources. A recent development of particular interest has been the production of food from unusual sources.

New foods may be developed by processing the proteins of plant foods which are in plentiful supply in such a way that they come to resemble foods such as meat. For example this has been done successfully with the soya bean, the original intention being to cater for the vegetarian market.

The soy flour is flavoured and coloured, then subjected to expansion and dehydration, the resulting product having a texture not unlike meat. An alternative, more elaborate process involves extraction of the proteins which are then spun into fibres as in the making of textiles. These fibres are then assembled to give an effect similar to that of meat. The latter product has a more realistic texture than the former but the process is more expensive.

The field bean is another example of a vegetable from which proteins have been extracted and subsequently processed by coagulation spinning.

These materials cannot of course be sold as meat and are known as textured vegetable protein products (TVP). They are used in the United Kingdom principally by manufacturers and caterers who include them, with meat, in composite dishes such as pies, as an economical means of supplementing the protein content. Nutritionally they stand comparison with other more conventional high-protein foods such as milk, eggs and beef.

Bacteria and yeasts can be grown in large quantities on suitable media. These include oil-refinery residues, and some companies, including Shell and B.P., have developed methods of growing micro-organisms in this way and then processing them to yield a food which has a high protein content and is a good source of vitamins of the B group. RHM Research Ltd. have developed a similar process, based on the growth of a micro-organism on carbohydrate.

Other unusual materials which are being considered as potential sources of protein include algae, plankton and leaves.

The development of a new food necessitates careful testing to ensure safety in all aspects of its use. The precise manner of its application must be determined, for example whether as food for animals or humans, and the manner of its incorporation into the diet. Food technology has advanced to the stage where there is a considerable range of possibilities.

The consumer must be assured of the suitability and safety of new foods. This is the responsibility of the Food Standards Committee of the Ministry of Agriculture, Fisheries and Food. The Ministry is at present reviewing several aspects of this field and has set up a novel protein intelligence unit. It would seem that we are about to become increasingly familiar with foods from unusual sources.

QUESTIONS

1. What nutrients does bread contain?
2. Which of these are important in the U.K. diet?
3. What differences in nutrient content are there between white and brown bread?
4. Which nutrients are provided by meat?
5. Vegetarians do not eat meat. Which foods should be included in their diet to compensate for this?

11

Conservation of food value; effect of cooking; some aspects of food production

SUMMARY

Food is only of value nutritionally if it is eaten. The cooking methods used should make the food palatable and appetising and retain as much of the nutritional value of the food as possible.

Cooking. The application of heat to food makes many foods more appetising and palatable, and easier and safer to eat. For example, raw meat looks unattractive, is unplatable and difficult to chew, but when properly cooked all these properties are changed. In an instance such as this cooking is beneficial. Food values, however, are sometimes impaired by cooking. In some cases flavours and nutrients are lost in water which is subsequently discarded. In other instances nutrients are rendered unavailable by chemical reactions which take place during preparation, cooking and serving. Yet again, food may be made unpalatable by poor cooking and incorrect seasoning. Ignorance of the effects of cooking procedures on foods results in a loss of nutritive value which may be greatly minimised by an intelligent appreciation of the factors involved.

CEREALS

Raw starch is insoluble in cold water. When cooked in an excess of water, as when cereals are used for thickening sauces and milk puddings, the starch granules swell and absorb water, and gelatinisation occurs.

When water is added to wheat flour, as in the making of bread, the proteins glutenin and gliadin combine to form gluten, which can be made to stretch and bring about expansion of the mixture. The expansion of the gluten is brought about by incorporating a raising agent. One such commonly employed is yeast, the growth of which in the dough results in the production of carbon dioxide gas. Chemical raising agents are also used. These consist of bicarbonate of soda in conjunction with an acid, such as cream of tartar or sour milk. They also give rise to the production of carbon dioxide in the dough. Air, incorporated during the preparation of the mixture, also acts as a raising agent, as does steam which is produced in the mixture during baking. The air, carbon dioxide or steam, or a combination of these, bring about expansion of the gluten, which is fixed by heat in this expanded position. Partial gelatinisation of the starch also occurs.

Dry heat converts starch to dextrins, which are intermediate products in the breakdown of the complex starch molecule to glucose and which are slightly sweet. Some caramel is also formed (see below). These changes take place when bread is toasted and in the crust of bread during baking, the brown appearance being due to the caramel.

During the baking of bread some loss of thiamin occurs and a further loss results from the use of chemical raising agents. The toasting of bread causes considerable loss of thiamin.

SUGAR

When a solution of sucrose (cane or loaf sugar) is boiled, some of the sucrose is converted to glucose and fructose. This process is called inversion and is assisted by the presence of acid, as is the case during jam-making and the stewing of fruits. The mixture of glucose and fructose thus formed is called invert sugar.

When sugar is heated to a high temperature it becomes brown in colour and develops a different flavour. This product is known as caramel and is used as a flavouring for puddings and as an ingredient of brownings used for colouring cakes and gravies.

VEGETABLES AND FRUITS

The cooking of vegetables softens their cellulose framework and makes then more easily masticated and more accessible to digestive enzymes. If the cooking water is discarded, the water-soluble vitamins and minerals which have been leached into it will also be lost. Fruit and vegetables are the only source of ascorbic acid in the diet. This nutrient is easily destroyed and care should be taken to preserve as much of it as possible. It is not unusual for 75 per cent of this vitamin to be lost.

Destruction of ascorbic acid

1. Ascorbic acid is oxidised by the oxygen in the atmosphere to an inactive form. This process is speeded up by light, heat and the metals, zinc, iron and copper.
2. Ascorbic acid is very soluble in water.
3. Plant cells contain the enzyme ascorbic acid oxidase which increases the rate of ascorbic acid oxidation. This enzyme is normally separated from the vitamin. However, if the plant cells are damaged by chopping, bruising or wilting, then the enzyme will come into contact with the ascorbic acid and it will be destroyed.
4. Ascorbic acid is unstable in alkaline conditions. Sodium bicarbonate is sometimes added to cooking vegetables to improve the colour which makes the cooking water alkaline and so destroys the ascorbic acid.

Steps necessary to minimise ascorbic acid losses

1. Use vegetables while they are fresh.
2. Prepare them immediately before cooking.
3. Use a sharp knife and if possible avoid peeling, grating and shredding.

4. Cook in boiling water as this destroys the enzyme ascorbic acid oxidase.
5. Use only a small amount of water.
6. Cook for the shortest possible time.
7. Have a lid on the saucepan.
8. If possible use the cooking water.
9. Serve immediately after cooking.

Some loss of vitamins occurs when vegetables are canned, dried or frozen. In general, losses resulting from drying are greater than from canning or freezing. At the same time vegetables prepared by modern methods retain much of their vitamin content, and can be superior to so-called fresh vegetables which have been kept in the kitchen until they are wilted, or which have been damaged by careless cooking and serving.

Fruits, like vegetables, are rendered more digestible by cooking, because of softening of the cellulose. Losses of ascorbic acid in cooking water are less important, as fruits, other than the citrus fruits, are not so important as a source of this vitamin as are vegetables, and in any case the juice is usually eaten along with the fruit.

Raw vegetables and fruits served in the form of salads introduce a variety of textures and flavours and add interest to meals. The food value of a salad is, of course, that of the ingredients used in its preparation. However, if the vegetables have been shredded, grated or stored, there will be a considerable loss of ascorbic acid.

FATS

When fats are heated to very high temperatures acrolein, a breakdown product of glycerol, is produced, which has an unpleasant acrid smell. Fat which is to be used for frying should be heated until a slight blue haze appears. A dense haze with an acrid odour indicates too high a temperature. On the other hand, if the fat is not hot enough to seal the surface of the food immediately the result will be greasy and unappetising. Fried foods are sometimes found to be indigestible, but this is frequently the result of faulty cooking.

Fats slow the rate of gastric emptying which can contribute to the feelings of nausea and fullness experienced in some disorders of the gastrointestinal tract. Fried foods always retain some of the cooking fat and so have a high energy content.

MEAT

Muscle meats consist of muscle fibres, connective tissue which holds the fibres together, and fat. The degree of tenderness of the meat depends upon the density of the connective tissue and the toughness of the muscle fibre. This in its turn is related to the age of the animal and the degree of activity associated with the particular cut. Thus lamb is more tender than mutton, and a cut such as the sirloin, from the back, is more tender than a section from the leg, which during life has been associated with much muscular activity. Deposits of fat within the muscle, giving a marbled appearance, are associated with the more tender cuts. Maturing or hanging of the carcase results in the formation of acids which assist the tenderising process.

Lengthy cooking is necessary to tenderise connective tissue, while the muscle fibres are hardened if high temperatures are used. Cooking of meat should aim at tenderising the connective tissue while avoiding as far as possible overcooking the muscle fibres.

Many different methods for cooking meat are used. The method which is chosen depends on the cut of meat, facilities available and personal preference of the cook.

Boiling and stewing. Heat is conducted from the water into the meat. Water soluble nutrients and flavour are lost into the water.

Pressure cooking. Heat is conducted into meat from the steam. Higher temperatures are reached, so cooking times can be shortened. Nutrients are lost into the cooking liquid.

Roasting and grilling. Convection from hot air and radiant heat cook the meat. As the meat shrinks, the juices are expelled and dry on the surface of the meat so fewer nutrients are lost.

Microwave cooking. This is a new method of cooking and is unusual because instead of applying heat to the food it is generated inside the food. The food is bombarded with electromagnetic radiation which causes the water molecules inside the food to oscillate. This oscillation generates heat energy which cooks the food. Because the food is not subject to direct heat it is not browned.

FISH

The flesh of fish is lacking in extractives and so lacks flavour when compared with meat, and the fibres tend to fall apart if it is overcooked or over handled during cooking. Care should be taken to prevent loss of flavouring ingredients in cooking water. the most conservative methods of cooking are steaming, grilling, frying, and poaching in milk which may be subsequently used in the preparation of a sauce. The more expensive fish, such as salmon, sole and halibut, have no nutritional advantages over the cheaper kinds, such as herrings and whiting.

MILK

Milk has a bland and unobtrusive flavour which does not pall on the appetite. This, along with its high nutritive value makes it a valuable food in illness.

When milk is heated in an uncovered pan a skin develops. This contains some of the protein, which is lost if the skin is discarded. This loss, however, is insignificant. A deposit also occurs on the sides and bottom of the pan. This, too, is protein in nature and tends to char, giving the milk a burnt flavour.

CHEESE

Cheese is a convenient high protein, high fat food, the nutritional content of which is unaltered by cooking.

EGGS

Eggs are a valuable food for sick persons as they are of high food value, are easily digested and can be incorporated into a large variety of attractive dishes, both savoury and sweet. Egg white coagulates at a temperature below boiling point and becomes toughened as the temperature increases.

SOME ASPECTS OF FOOD PRODUCTION

The continual evolution of new and improved methods of agriculture and food processing is essential to the feeding of a world population which is increasing rapidly. Some examples of developments which have benefited mankind are the use of pesticides, the introduction of inorganic fertilisers, the intensive rearing of livestock, and the use of antibiotics in animal husbandry. We have also seen the introduction of radiation as a means of food preservation. New sources of food are being investigated; some of these are discussed in Chapter 10.

Developments such as these require careful study in order to ensure the maximum benefit to mankind and to reduce potential health hazards to the minimum. For example pesticides help to secure maximum crop yields. Some of them, however, remain in the crop after harvesting and processing and are eventually found in food. Small amounts of pesticide residues can be detected in human fat and the result of long-term ingestion of this material is not yet known. Some pesticides have come under suspicion and have been withdrawn from use.

Antibiotics are used in the treatment of infectious diseases in livestock. If recommended procedures are not followed on the farm this may give rise to residues in foodstuffs. For example milk containing a trace of penicillin has been known to cause reactions in already-sensitised persons, although such cases are rare.

Certain antibiotics have been found to accelerate growth, for example in broiler fowls and in pigs, and for this reason have been used as components of feeding mixtures. Statutory control is exercised over which antibiotics are permitted and how much may be fed. So far there is little evidence to suggest that this practice gives rise to harmful residues in foods derived from these animals.

Many of the foods we eat contain additives, for example preservatives, colouring or flavouring agents, or emulsifiers. Careful control is exercised, and enforced by legislation where necessary, otherwise toxic materials, including possible carcinogens, could be introduced into the diet in this way.

Developments such as these must be considered in the light of expected benefits and any risks taken must be calculated ones. It is also relevant to note that certain foods which we eat regularly, and which we take entirely for granted, contain harmful material; for example the goitrogens present in members of the cabbage family (p. 83), the toxic substance solanin which is found in potatoes, and oxalic acid which is present in rhubarb. Fluorine, a constituent of water and important for the development of teeth which are resistant to decay, produces harmful effects if present in excessive amounts. The taking of food in fact, has never been free from hazard.

It is not surprising that the food industry is deeply involved in experiment and research and that the application of food technology requires careful judgement and control. Bodies concerned in this work represent the government, the food industry, and scientific disciplines such as medicine. The Ministry of Agriculture, Fisheries and Food has various bodies monitoring food, for example the Steering Group on Food Surveillance, the Working Party on the Monitoring of Foodstuffs for Heavy Metals, and the Panel for the Collection of Residues Data. In the international field the Codex Alimentarius Commission, set up by FAO and WHO, promotes co-ordination of food standards. It may be said that our food has never been so carefully scrutinised as at present.

It is not proposed within the scope of this book to discuss the subject of food technology in detail. The nurse is referred to the suggestions for further reading on page 296, in particular to the journal *Nutrition and Food Science*, and the Information Bulletins of the British Nutrition Foundation.

In these publications the subject is dealt with in a simple manner by experts. By keeping herself informed the nurse can use her influence in the community to counteract the propaganda of the scaremongers and food faddists who crave for a return to 'natural' foods, or preach the magical properties of molasses, honey and wheat germ.

QUESTIONS

1. How should vegetables be cooked in order to preserve their ascorbic acid content?
2. Why does overcooking make some meat tough?
3. Many foods contain additives. List three and explain why they are necessary.

12

Food-borne diseases and their prevention

SUMMARY

Food, although essential for life, may produce illness if it contains harmful bacteria or parasites, or poisonous chemicals. Care is needed in all stages of food preparation to ensure that the food is uncontaminated and will not cause illness.

BACTERIA IN FOOD

Most species of bacteria are not harmful to man and many perform useful functions. Examples of these are the lactic acid bacteria which ferment lactose with the production of lactic acid and thus bring about the souring of milk. These bacteria play a part in the ripening of cheese and are also responsible for the production of fermented milks such as yoghurt. Other examples are the bacteria which synthesise vitamins in the intestine, and the bacteria of the soil, which break down waste material and convert it to plant foodstuffs.

Some bacteria, however, are pathogenic, that is to say they can cause disease. These pathogenic species demand our attention as some may be taken into the body along with food and may give rise to illness. It is important to know how food becomes infected with these bacteria and what precautions should be taken to guard against such infection.

Food poisoning

The term food poisoning is applied to acute inflammation of the gastrointestinal tract following the consumption of food which contains harmful material. The condition may be caused by ingestion of poisonous articles such as certain berries and fungi, or food contaminated with chemical poisons such as lead or zinc, but the most common cause by far is the infection of food by pathogenic bacteria. Sometimes the food is infected at the source, as in the case of meat from a diseased animal. Alternatively infection may take place during handling of the food if certain precautions to be discussed later are not observed.

Food poisoning bacteria

Certain bacteria of the Salmonella group are well known as a cause of food poisoning. These bacteria may remain in the intestinal tract of infected persons for some time after recovery has taken place. Such persons are said to be carriers and may, through faulty personal hygiene, be the means of spreading the disease.

Cooked meat which has been handled by a person suffering from the condition or who is a carrier is a common source of infection. Other foods concerned in salmonella food poisoning include meat or milk from infected animals, and milk and milk foods infected by a food handler. Eggs can be a source of salmonella infection. Flies may be the means of spreading the disease. Rats and mice are particularly susceptible to salmonella infections and may transmit the disease to man by contamination of food with excreta.

These bacteria are destroyed by thorough cooking. They like moisture and warmth, and provided the medium is suitable will multiply rapidly in food which is being kept warm for some time before being eaten.

Certain strains of staphylococci are also known to cause food poisoning. The symptoms are brought about as a result of the ingestion of a toxic substance formed by the bacteria during their period of growth in the food. This substance is referred to as an enterotoxin because of its effect on the gastrointestinal tract.

Common sources of infection are (1) septic conditions such as boils and abscesses in people concerned with the handling of food—such lesions harbour staphylococci which are transmitted to the food from the hands of the infected person; (2) respiratory infections in food handlers, the organisms being transmitted to the food from the hands, or directly in droplets discharged from the respiratory tract as in speaking or coughing. Food poisoning staphylococci may also be present in the respiratory tract and on the skin of healthy persons.

Staphylococcal food poisoning is associated with foods which have been infected during preparation and have then been set aside for some hours before being eaten. During this period the bacteria grow in the food and the toxin is produced. Such foods include meats such as ham, tongue, meat pies and brawn, and to a lesser extent milk and milk dishes and artificial cream.

Staphylococci are destroyed by cooking, but this is not always true of the enterotoxin.

Clostridium perfringens may also give rise to food poisoning. These organisms are present in soil and are normal inhabitants of the intestines of both animals and humans. From these sources food becomes infected. These bacteria form spores, of which those of the food poisoning variety may survive cooking. Meat is a particularly favourite medium for growth. when a large quantity of meat is cooked at one time heat penetration may be insufficient to kill the spores, which later germinate and multiply if the food is not eaten at once, but allowed to cool. The poisoning is due to a toxin which the bacteria produce while they multiply in the intestine.

Another food poisoning organism is *Bacillus cereus* which is found in a variety of foods, especially cereals. This form of food poisoning had been associated particularly with rice served in Chinese restaurants. The organism forms spores which can survive cooking. The rice is parboiled some hours before it is required and kept at room temperature, during which time the spores germinate and produce a toxin in the food. The final frying of the rice prior to serving is insufficient to destroy the toxin which is subsequently ingested, resulting in food poisoning. Prevention necessitates reducing the interval between parboiling and frying to less than two hours. Rice should be parboiled in small batches, cooled quickly, and kept in a refrigerator.

In the United Kingdom, food poisoning bacteria of the Salmonella group are responsible for a high proportion of all recorded outbreaks. Next in importance are the staphylococci and *Cl. perfringens*. Other organisms have been shown to be responsible to a lesser degree for food poisoning. In many recorded outbreaks the organisms responsible have not been identified.

The following quotation from *Bacterial Food Poisoning** demonstrates the importance of meat as a vehicle of infection in food poisoning outbreaks.

Associated foods

'Between 1949 and 1966 there were about 3800 general and family outbreaks . . . in which there was reasonable certainty that the food concerned had been identified.

Of these outbreaks:

75 per cent were associated with meat
8 per cent with sweetmeats
5 per cent with fish
5 per cent with egg and egg products
3 per cent with milk and milk products
2 per cent with vegetables
1 per cent with fruit
and 1 per cent with other foods.'

Some other diseases resulting from bacterial infection of food

Tuberculosis and brucellosis (undulant fever) may be transmitted by milk, the original source of the infection being the udder of the cow.

Bovine tuberculosis has been almost totally eradicated from the United Kingdom. Brucellosis eradication programmes are being implemented. In Great Britain around 90 per cent of

---

* From W. C. Cockburn and E. Vernon (1969). Reporting and incidence of food poisoning. In *Bacterial Food Poisoning*, ed. J. Taylor. London: The Royal Society of Health.

herds are brucellosis free. In Northern Ireland, where herds are smaller, almost 100 per cent are free from the disease. In the United Kingdom as a whole approximately 97 per cent of milk sold in liquid form is pasteurised. The relatively small number of people drinking milk prior to pasteurisation, or drinking farm-bottled milk, are at risk of contracting undulant fever depending upon the position in their particular area. Other infections of cattle may be transmitted by means of raw milk, for example salmonellosis and Q fever.

Typhoid fever and paratyphoid fever are often associated with poor sewage disposal resulting in contaminated water supply. Oysters and other shell-fish may be a source of typhoid bacteria if they have been obtained from water which is contaminated with sewage. In the United Kingdom, legislation relating to the gathering and sale of shell-fish helps to prevent the spread of infection in this way.

Botulism is a serious and often fatal disease of rare occurrence in the United Kingdom. It results from the ingestion of a toxin produced by the bacterium *Clostridium botulinum*. This organism is present in soil. Vegetables, fruit, meat and fish are susceptible to infection. The bacteria multiply in food in the absence of oxygen and the toxin is a product of their growth. In adverse conditions they develop spores, in which form they are able to survive until conditions once more become favourable for growth. The toxin is destroyed by heat but the spores are heat resistant, requiring very high temperatures to destroy them.

No harm would result from the ingestion of infected food while fresh, but in the case of canned or bottled food, if sterilising procedures have not been correctly carried out spores may survive, in which case finding conditions in the can favourable for growth they subsequently multiply in the food, rendering it poisonous.

The spores are more heat-resistant in non-acid foods such as carrots, peas, beans and most vegetables than in the acid conditions associated with some fruits. Persons interested in home canning or bottling of fruit and vegetables should obtain reliable advice and follow it explicity. Manufacturers of canned meats and other susceptible foods exercise great care, and foods heat-processed commercially may be considered safe.

PARASITIC INFESTATION

Food which contains animal parasites can be a means of transmitting these to humans. Tapeworm infestation can result from eating beef or pork which contains the organisms in the form of cysts. The cysts are destroyed by thorough cooking of the meat.

The eggs of roundworms and threadworms may be present on food which is contaminated with human faeces. These also are destroyed during cooking. This type of infestation is particularly liable to occur in countries where crops are fertilised with human excreta.

CHEMICALS IN FOODS

Poisoning may result from the presence in food of chemicals, traces of which are not necessarily harmful, but which could be harmful if present in sufficient quantity.

We have already seen, in Chapter 9, that traces of pesticides used in agriculture can remain in the crop after harvesting, that antibiotics given to animals could possibly be present in animal products in significant amount, and that many foods contain chemical additives which are necessary for technical or other reasons.

Traces of lead are present in many foods in amounts which are not harmful. However certain specific foods have a greater than normal lead content. Plumbing systems still in use in some older houses contribute lead to the water. Certain plastic packaging material, in direct contact with the food, can leave a residue.

In this highly technical age, governments must be on the alert. In the United Kingdom the presence of these and other chemicals in food is constantly monitored, and such matters as the presence of a particular material in a specific food, whether or not it is potentially harmful, the amount likely to be ingested, and the setting of safe limits are the responsibility of bodies such as the Steering Group on Food Surveillance of the Food Science Division of the Ministry of Agriculture, Fisheries and Food. The Government has powers under the Food and Drugs Act of 1955, to make and enforce

Regulations when these are necessary, to ensure safe food for the consumer.

In the home, chemicals such as weed-killers and cleaning materials may be added to food in error. It is the responsibility of every individual to exercise care in the labelling and storage of such material.

FOOD SAFETY

National legislation sets compulsory standards for the production, distribution and sale of foodstuffs, and provides local authorities with the power to make by-laws to meet the special needs of each area. For example control is exercised over the circumstances in which milk may be produced or distributed, and there are standards with regard to bacteriological contamination to which all milk sold for human consumption must conform. Animals intended for slaughter must be free from disease, and carcases are subject to inspection. There are specifications covering the handling, wrapping and sale of foods, and premises used for the sale of food or the production of food intended for sale must conform to certain specifications. Control is exercised over the addition of chemicals to foods, for example as preservatives or as colouring matter.

It will be seen, then, that legislation relating to the production and distribution of foodstuffs affords a very considerable degree of protection to the consumer. It should be appreciated, however, that legislation is of necessity limited in its scope, and that its ultimate effectiveness depends upon the co-operation of each individual concerned in food-handling.

Guidance for the food-handler

Food may be heavily contaminated with pathogenic organisms and yet show no visible signs of spoilage, being unaffected in appearance, odour or taste.

Poisonous chemicals may easily be mistaken for foods and used as such if tins and bottles are not labelled, or if both are kept in the same store cupboard. The presence of such poisonous material in food may be unsuspected until the food has been sampled and then, probably, the damage will have been done.

It will be seen, therefore, that food which appears in every way wholesome may yet contain pathogenic organisms or other harmful material. Safety depends upon the adoption of safe methods of handling food. The following rules should be observed:

1. Wash the hands before preparing food and cover lesions such as cuts and burns with waterproof dressings.

2. Wash the hands after blowing the nose or going to the toilet; do not allow persons with septic skin conditions, respiratory infections or diarrhoea to handle food.

3. Do not touch food with the fingers unnecessarily.

4. See that food is protected from rats, mice, flies and domestic pets.

5. Do not leave crumbs and food particles lying around the kitchen; keep refuse bins covered.

6. Keep foods which provide good media for multiplication of bacteria in as cool a place as possible, as low temperatures inhibit bacterial growth, a refrigerator is ideal for this purpose.

7. The refrigerator must be cleaned regularly and its contents checked.

8. Avoid partial cooking of joints of meat intended for use on the following day, as this results in a temperature in the centre, favourable to bacterial growth. A similar effect occurs in frozen chickens if these have not been completely thawed before cooking.

9. Do not attempt to assess the condition of suspected food by tasting it. This practice is both dangerous and ineffectual.

10. Store chemicals such as insecticides, cleaning materials and medicines away from food, and out of the reach of children. See that containers are clearly labelled.

QUESTION

What precautions must be taken in a ward kitchen to prevent food poisoning?

13

Dietary recommendations for adults

SUMMARY

Good nutrition is essential for health. An inadequate diet causes dietary deficiency disease. The diet of affluent Western man is associated with the increased incidence of some diseases.

The dietary changes recommended to combat this are the increased consumption of starchy fibre-rich foods (bread, fruit and vegetables) and a decrease in the consumption of sugar, fat, salt and alcohol.

INTRODUCTION

Most of us choose food we like rather than the food which is best for our health.

This quotation is taken from the Foreword of the DHSS publication *Eating for Health* and states the problem succinctly. The nutritional value of food is not the major influence governing the food choices of most people. Their choice is influenced by cost and availability of food, by their culture and by personal preferences. Any attempt to change dietary habits is difficult because long standing preferences and opinions must be overcome. For dietary advice to be effective it must be both practical and acceptable. The best way to achieve this is to base advice on simple modifications of existing habits. It is both impractical and unreasonable to expect anyone, except in the most extreme situations, to adopt a completely new diet.

It is now well established that diet has an important part in maintaining health and in the prevention of disease. It also has an important role in the treatment of disease. Preceding chapters of this book have treated nutrients as separate entities. In this chapter general nutritional advice is given which applies to all adults. More specific nutritional advice for groups with special nutritional needs, such as the elderly and immigrants, is given in other chapters.

Recommended daily intakes

Tables of the Recommended Daily Intake (or Recommended Daily Allowance) for a variety of nutrients are published in many countries.

The recommended daily intake is the average amount of a nutrient required per day to provide for the needs of a healthy person. It is enough to maintain normal metabolic balance and prevent the development of disease. Requirements in disease are different. The recommended daily amounts of food energy and nutrients for groups of people in the U.K., published by DHSS (Report by the Committee on Medical Aspects of Food Policy of the Department of Health and Social Security: Report on Health and Social Subjects *15*, 1979) are reproduced in Appendix 2. They are not intended to be used rigidly as a guide to an individual's diet because individual dietary requirements vary greatly. They are used as a reference point in population nutritional surveys, in planning food supplies, and in large scale catering operations in institutions.

Dietary guidelines

Recommended daily intakes cannot be used for individual diet planning. To overcome this problem, Government committees were appointed in Sweden, Norway, Canada, USA, Ireland, France and the U.K. to prepare individual national nutritional guidelines. They reviewed the enormous amount of research into diet and disease, much of which was conflicting, and produced reports which provide a consensus of informed opinion that can be acted upon by all those concerned with food, nutrition and health. These include food manufacturers, teachers, health workers and the public. All seven reports agreed that the incidence of obesity must be reduced and that diets should be modified to contain less sugar and fat and more fibre and starch. Some reports also recommended a reduction in salt intake, alcohol consumption and the amount of cholesterol in the diet, and an increase in the proportion of fat from polyunsaturated sources. Others felt that the evidence for this was inconclusive. The ten recommendations of the DHSS report are printed in Appendix 3 and those concerned with adult nutrition are explained below.

Reduce average intake of total fat

Fat is the most concentrated form of energy in the diet, a reduction in fat intake would reduce the energy content of the diet and so prevent, in some cases, the development of obesity. A high dietary fat intake will probably raise blood lipid levels, which are associated with increased risk of coronary artery disease. There is also epidemiological evidence that links a high fat diet with an increased incidence of breast and colonic cancer.

Reduce average intake of sugar and increase intake of starch and dietary fibre

Refined sugar contributes about 20 per cent of the daily energy intake. It provides energy and contains no other nutrients such as vitamins and minerals. It causes dental caries and may be linked to coronary artery disease. Sugar and sugary food should be replaced with unrefined starchy carbohydrate foods such as bread, potatoes, fruit and vegetables. These foods are rich sources of a variety of nutrients, such as minerals and vitamins and also contain dietary fibre. The increased incidence of many diseases in developed countries has developed as the diet has become increasingly fibre-depleted.

Reduce average salt intake

The dietary salt intake of most people exceeds their physiological requirement. The major source of salt is in processed foods. One of the factors that raises blood pressure in some people is a high salt intake. A reduction in salt intake would be beneficial for this group.

Reduce average alcohol intake

Alcohol is high in calories and is not a necessary food. Excessive alcohol intake causes cirrhosis of the liver, pancreatitis and is linked to increased incidence of carcinoma of oesophagus and stomach and coronary artery disease.

The DHSS report was criticised by some groups because it did not give quantitative advice about the nutritional content of the diet. In 1979 Passmore, Hollingsworth and Robertson published dietary recommendations which were related to the average British diet. The values for the average intake of food were obtained from the National Food Survey. The improvements recommended are listed below.

Decreased consumption of:

Fats and oils	by 15 per cent
Sugar	by 15 per cent
Meat	by 15 per cent
Alcohol	by 25 per cent

Increased consumption of:

Potatoes	by 15 per cent
Other vegetables	by 15 per cent
Fruit	by 15 per cent
Grain products	by 20 per cent

The net result of these changes is an improvement in the overall nutritional quality of the national diet. The energy, protein, fat and carbohydrate content of the average British diet and the new target figures for a 'Better British Diet' are listed in Table 13.1. These figures are for the average national diet. It is impossible to give a precise recommendation for the ideal diet because of the enormous inter-individual variations in nutritional requirement.

Table 13.1 Nutrient content of the British diet, figures are expressed as a percentage of total energy intake

	Carbohydrate	Fat	Protein	Alcohol
Average British diet	46.0	38.0	11.0	5.0
Better British diet	50.0	35.0	11.0	4.0

MEAL PLANNING

It is only in large institutions that meals are planned by calculation of their nutrient content. They are generally planned to provide a palatable mixture of foods. A knowledge of nutrition is of little value if it is not translated into practical terms. For example, choosing baked potatoes instead of chips will increase the fibre content and decrease the fat content of a meal. The DHSS dietary guidelines can be implemented in the following ways.

1. Eat a variety of foods. This ensures that the diet contains adequate amounts of all nutrients.
2. Reduce sugar intake by eating fewer cakes, sweets and biscuits and by drinking unsweetened beverages.
3. Increase the fibre and starch content of the diet by eating more bread, potatoes, cereal products, fruit and vegetables.
4. Reduce the salt content of the diet by not relying on processed foods and not seasoning food excessively.
5. Reduce fat intake by cutting off fat from meat, eating less butter, margarine and cream, and by grilling food instead of frying it.

If the meals for a day include two portions of protein-rich foods such as meat, fish, egg or pulses, three portions of wholegrain cereals, two portions of fresh fruit or vegetables, half a pint of milk and a small amount of fat, the diet will be nutritionally adequate.

Convenience foods

The range of convenience foods available is constantly

increasing as the food industry identifies new markets and develops new products. They can be divided into two groups.
1. Ready prepared forms of food which are traditionally eaten as part of a main meal e.g., instant mashed potato, frozen peas, ready made pies.
2. New foods which are intended as snack meals or between meal snacks e.g., instant dehydrated meals, potato crisps, quick soups.

Many of the foods in the first group have become established as part of our national diet and add variety and interest to it. The freezing of vegetables ensures a wide range of good quality products throughout the year. It is usual for a convenience food, which in its traditional form is an important source of a particular nutrient, to be enriched with that nutrient. Examples are replacement of vitamin C lost in processing in potatoes, and fortification of soya meat substitutes with iron and B vitamins. As a general rule, convenience products have a high sugar and salt content. This is particularly so for tinned foods. However, as more families own refrigerators and freezers they rely on frozen instead of tinned foods, the nutritional content of which is high. All cakes, biscuits, pies and puddings have a high sugar content irrespective of whether they are home made or bought.

Foods which belong to the second group are of less value nutritionally. They provide carbohydrate, fat, salt and sugar and their instant preparation makes them convenient. However, although useful, they should not be relied upon as sources of essential nutrients other than energy.

'Take away' meals. In the last ten years there has been an increase in both the type and number of 'take away' restaurants and they are increasing in popularity particularly with the under 30 age group. The food chosen from 'Take aways' is usually different to that prepared at home and is often considered 'junk food'. It is possible to choose well-balanced meals by avoiding deep fried foods and including salads.

Some adults in the population have special nutritional needs, either because of restrictions they impose on their diet e.g. vegetarians, or because of their increased need, e.g. pregnant and lactating women. The nutritional requirements of both these groups are included in this chapter.

Dietary requirements during pregnancy and lactation

The requirements for most nutrients are increased during pregnancy and lactation. Weight gain occurs during pregnancy due to the increase in size of the reproductive tissues, the foetus and the maternal fat stores. During her pregnancy a woman will gain about 12.5 kg in weight, 3.5 kg of this will be in the first 20 weeks and then the rate is about 0.5 kg per week. If a pregnant woman's diet is varied and provides adequate energy for sufficient weight gain, the increased requirements of most nutrients will be met. Additional milk is recommended to provide the extra calcium required during the third trimester and during lactation—500 ml a day is the recommended amount. During pregnancy routine supplements of iron and folic acid are prescribed.

Vegetarian diets

The nutritional problems of immigrants who are vegetarians are discussed in Chapter 15. There are three types of vegetarians and each type has a different dietary restriction.

Type of vegetarian	*Diet*
1. Total vegetarian (Vegan)	Plant foods only
2. Lacto-vegetarian	Plant foods and dairy produce
3. Lacto-ovo-vegetarian	Plant foods, dairy products and eggs

Vegetarians do not eat meat and have a variety of reasons for this. Religious beliefs and moral views are important, some people dislike meat whilst others cannot afford it. Meat is an expensive and inefficient source of food to produce, 30 kg of cattle food is needed to produce 1 kg of beef.

Vegetarian diets can be nutritionally adequate as long as care is taken in their planning. The diets of lacto-vegetarians and lacto-ovo-vegetarians do not lead to nutritional deficiencies whilst the Vegan diet contains marginal amounts of calcium, iron, riboflavin and vitamin B12. Fortified soya products need to be included in the diet to supplement the small amount of calcium, iron and riboflavin provided by green vegetables. Plant foods do not contain vitamin B12 and a supplement is necessary either by injection or from a soya milk which has been fortified. Not all vegetarian milks are suitable for children and if a child is not breast fed, care is needed to ensure that the substitute milk provides adequate supplies of all nutrients.

Other nutritional deficiencies can occur among vegetarians if food supplies are limited or dietary intake is restricted. Vegetarian meals are bulky and should have a mixture of pulses and cereals and large helpings of fruit and vegetables to be satisfactory.

Two advantages accompany a vegetarian diet. These are that obesity is rare and serum cholesterol is usually low in vegetarians. However, whether this is due to the exclusion of meat or the increased amounts of pulses, cereals and vegetables is uncertain.

Vegetarians often include organically produced food in their diet. This is food which has been produced without the addition of chemical pesticides and fertilisers.

Cult diets and food fads which restrict the variety of foods eaten are particularly harmful to children who have relatively high requirements for all nutrients.

CONCLUSION

Diets can be modified to provide the optimum amounts of nutrients for health. This is done by including a wide range of foods in the diet and by choosing low fat, low sugar, high fibre carbohydrate sources.

QUESTIONS

1. Why should less sugar be eaten?
2. Suggest three ways in which fat intake can be reduced.
3. Plan a 'healthy' menu for two days.
4. a. Which nutritional deficiencies is a Vegan likely to suffer from?
   b. How can the diet be modified to prevent this?

14

Nutrition and the elderly

SUMMARY

Improvements in public health and new developments in medical knowledge have led to a dramatic increase in life expectancy. Sixteen per cent of the population of the United Kingdom are now over retirement age.

Nutritional deficiencies occur in the over 75 age group and are usually associated with a social, medical or physical problem. Much can be done to prevent the development of nutritional deficiencies in the elderly.

INTRODUCTION

> When, like a running grave, time tracks you down.
> Dylan Thomas

Although many long for retirement, few look forward to old age. It is seen as a time when, with failing faculties, people are no longer able to live useful independent lives. This is an unfortunate but understandable attitude. Most people are perfectly able to cope within their limitations until they are well into their eighth decade.

It is not surprising that many products are sold which claim to prevent or slow the aging process. Some products are based on folklore and herbalism, for example, honey and cider vinegar; some, such as ginseng, are based on the mystique of the Orient; whilst others—large doses of vitamins—are based on distorted scientific fact. However, most people believe that their diet will in some way influence their allotted life span. This is particularly true for people who become centenarians who, when interviewed, will claim that their diet contributed to their longevity. However, there is no particular diet that they all claim has benefited them. Each person has his particular 'pet' food and also particular foods which he considers harmful and has avoided. There is rarely any logical basis for any of these prejudices.

The elderly population

Infection, disease and accidents, combined with the gradual degenerative processes, cause death for most of the population. The maximum age for man is said to be 110 years. Very few people approach this age. As medical treatment improves and death as a result of infection, disease and accidents becomes less likely, the population lives longer. The figures for the number of people over retirement age in this country show the dramatic effect of improved medical services and better standards of living. In 1901 there were 2.4 million people over retirement age, this being 6 per cent of the total population. This figure has now quadrupled to 10 million and, more importantly, the percentage of the total population has increased to 16 per cent. The increase obviously places more demands on the health and social services.

The size of this section of the population is no longer increasing but the age distribution within the group is changing. More people now live longer. It has been predicted that the number of people in the 75–85 year age group will have increased by a third by the year 1990. This will put even greater demands on the already stretched services. It is in this age group that the incidences of disease, disability and malnutrition are highest.

Meat - 1 portion
2 eggs - 1 portion

The aging process

This process starts once growth is complete at the age of 25. Few people are aware that it has started (apart from the odd grey hair!) and it causes no problems. Later on these processes speed up and physiological changes become apparent. It is not always easy to distinguish between the frailty caused by physiological changes and the physical decline which accompanies malnutrition. These degenerative changes include:

> Loss of sensations of smell and taste
> Deafness
> Failing sight
> Osteoarthritis
> Osteoporosis
> Arterial disease
> Reduction of glucose tolerance
> Decline in muscle bulk and strength

Little can be done to prevent these, except perhaps avoiding obesity. Extra weight makes mobility difficult and more painful for arthritis sufferers; it impairs glucose tolerance and is a contributory cause of the development of arterial disease.

Nutritional requirements of the elderly

The nutritional requirements of the elderly are the same as those of the younger population: the only exception to this being a fall in energy requirement with age. The reasons for this are:

1. Activity declines with age, so less energy is expended.
2. Changes in body composition and function lead to a reduction in basal metabolic rate.

Figure 14.1 shows the changes in energy requirement for men that occur with age. There is a similar change for women. Their energy requirement drops from 2200 kcal (9.2 MJ) at the age of 18, to 1900 kcal (8.0 MJ) at the age of 75.

The practical implications of this reduction are:

1. Unless energy intake is reduced body weight will increase.
2. The diet has to be of a high nutritional quality to ensure

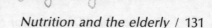

1g Protein per Kg of body weight.
1g " - 4 Kcal
1g Carb. - " " "
1g 70

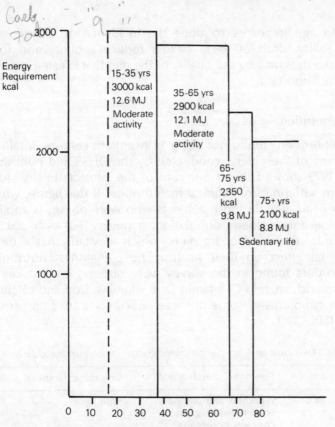

Energy Requirement kcal

15-35 yrs
3000 kcal
12.6 MJ
Moderate activity

35-65 yrs
2900 kcal
12.1 MJ
Moderate activity

65-75 yrs
2350 kcal
9.8 MJ

75+ yrs
2100 kcal
8.8 MJ
Sedentary life

Figure 14.1 Change in energy requirement with age for men.

that the requirements for all other nutrients are met, whilst the energy intake (total amount of food) eaten is reduced.

Certain individuals in the elderly population have increased requirements of certain nutrients. This is not a problem that is specific to the elderly. It occurs in any group of people but more commonly in the elderly. For example, the housebound elderly require more dietary vitamin D. The recommended intake for the elderly who are not housebound is 2.5 µg cholecalciferol a day. The current recommendation for the housebound is 10 µg a day.

Those elderly people who are immobilised, have bed sores or prolonged fevers, will have an increased nitrogen requirement and require more protein to prevent a negative nitrogen balance (see Ch. 21, Diet and Injury).

Reduce Protein during Renal failure

As age increases so does the incidence of disease and disability. Both of these factors reduce appetite and food intake thus making the quality of the diet that is eaten increasingly important.

Malnutrition

Malnutrition should not occur in twentieth century Britain. A survey of the elderly conducted by the DHSS and published in 1979 showed that 3 per cent of the subjects in the study were suffering from clinical malnutrition. If this figure, which does not include those subjects who were obese, is applied to the entire elderly population, it means that over 300 000 people have inadequate diets, which inevitably has a detrimental effect on their health. The commonest nutritional disorders found in the survey were obesity, low intakes of folic acid, vitamin C, vitamin D, B vitamins, iron and calcium. The symptoms of some of these deficiencies are summarised in Table 14.1.

Table 14.1 Nutritional deficiencies which occur in some of the elderly

Nutrient	Symptoms of deficiency	Easy dietary sources
Vitamin C	Weakness and tiredness Sore, bleeding gums Poor wound healing	Fruit juice
Vitamin D	Osteomalacia Bone pain Spontaneous fractures Low serum calcium	(Sunshine) Fortified margarines and milk products
Folic acid	Megaloblastic anaemia Tiredness and lassitude Inflamed red tongue	Green vegetables Yeast extracts
Iron	Hypochromic anaemia Tiredness Headaches Brittle, spoon-shaped nails Sore tongue	Meat

The malnourished elderly can be divided into three groups.
1. Generalised malnutrition. The diet contains inadequate supplies of several nutrients. This is due to generalised self-neglect which is caused by a wide variety of circumstances.

2. Deficiency of a particular nutrient. This occurs when a particular food or group of foods is excluded from the diet. Two examples are: iron deficiency in those with poor teeth who avoid meat because it needs chewing; and low vitamin C intake in those who were prescribed a 'gastric diet' long ago and still keep to it.

3. Obesity. The magnitude of this problem increases if energy intake is not reduced as activity decreases. It is unusual for extreme obesity to develop after retirement. Obesity is usually due to a lifetime of bad eating habits. It is important to be aware of the disadvantages of being obese in later life. Mobility becomes more difficult. The tasks of nursing and rehabilitating the obese are difficult.

Sub-clinical malnutrition

A large group of the elderly suffer from sub-clinical malnutrition. This means that their diet is not so poor that they show the clinical features of malnutrition but that their body stores of nutrients are depleted. If exposed to any sort of stress that reduces their dietary intake or increases their requirements, this group is likely to become clinically malnourished. They are inevitably a group at higher risk of developing other diseases.

Causes of malnutrition in the elderly (summarised in Table 14.2)

Malnutrition is rarely the only problem of an elderly person. Malnutrition does not usually occur in isolation but is precipitated by other social, physical or medical problems.

Extreme age. The increasing frailty of extreme old age increases the risks of malnutrition.

Social isolation and loneliness. Fourteen per cent of the elderly live alone. As life expectancy increases this percentage will also increase. It is easy to understand why people living alone cannot be bothered to cook for themselves. Meal times are particularly lonely for the recently bereaved. The importance of social contact to the wellbeing of the elderly must never be underestimated. The practical problems of catering for one are also difficult. It is hard to find small portions of

Table 14.2 Causes of malnutrition in the elderly

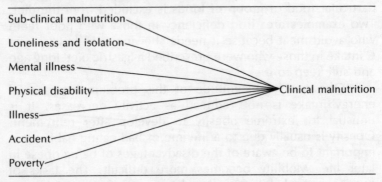

Sub-clinical malnutrition
Loneliness and isolation
Mental illness
Physical disability
Illness
Accident
Poverty

Clinical malnutrition

fresh food, especially meat. The elderly will often avoid eating meat rather than be embarassed in the butcher's shop by asking for one lamb chop. Pre-retirement courses (mentioned at the end of the chapter) are a very successful way of introducing new methods of cooking and types of food that are suitable for a single person. They also provide an opportunity to discuss the changing dietary requirements of retirement and later life.

Loss of appetite. Anyone who listens to the radio programme 'Gardeners' Question Time' will know that one of the questions most frequently asked is 'Why don't fruit and vegetables taste like they did 20 years ago?' The answer lies both with the gardener or the cook and with the consumer. Market pressures have led the food industry to produce foods which keep better and look more attractive at the expense of flavour and texture. It is also true that the questioner's sense of taste and smell have deteriorated. This loss of appreciation of food, accompanied by loss of appetite, means that less food is eaten. There are numerous causes for loss of appetite. In the elderly, reduced activity, illness and certain drug treatments are all important.

Ignorance. Most ideas about food and dietary preferences develop in childhood. Attitudes formed 70 years ago are difficult to change. However, a survey conducted in Surrey has shown that the elderly can change their eating habits with suitable encouragement. This means that nutrition education is important both before and after retirement. Many women have deeply held prejudices about the values and uses of

certain foods. Convenience foods are frequently discounted as rubbish, although many of these foods are as nutritious as their freshly prepared counterparts and could add easy variety to the diet.
Examples of convenience foods which can usefully be included in the diet of the elderly.
Frozen vegetables
'Boil in the bag meals' e.g. fish in sauce
Instant mashed potato
Tinned milk puddings
Widowers who were never allowed by their wives to cook a meal are a particularly vulnerable group. They are usually unaware of the values of a well-balanced diet. They are often ill-prepared to shop, plan and prepare their own meals. The plight of men in this group has led to the term 'widower's disease' being applied to vitamin C deficiency. A man aged 75 and living alone is four times as likely to have a low dietary intake of vitamin C than a man of the same age who lives with his wife or family.

Mental disturbances. Senile dementia affects 5 per cent of the post-retirement population. People in this group often forget to prepare or eat meals. Elderly people who are isolated often become depressed and apathetic. They cannot be bothered to shop for, prepare or eat meals. The local services of lunch clubs, day centres and meals on wheels are very important in improving the nutrition of this group.

Physical disability. Ten per cent of the elderly are housebound because of physical disability. In the elderly these include hemiplegia, arthritis, Parkinson's disease and injuries from accidents. If the sufferer can be encouraged to try, much can be done to overcome the problems in catering which handicaps cause. Home helps can do the shopping and occupational therapists can recommend aids for the kitchen such as specially adapted utensils which make meal preparation easier. For the group of very disabled elderly who are in residential care, food must be provided which can be eaten easily and yet looks appetising. A boiled egg is very difficult to eat with only one hand!

Poverty: '. . . and I shall spend my pension on brandy, summer gloves and satin sandals, and say we've no money for butter'
Jenny Joseph

This sort of mismanagement is rarely the cause of a poor diet. Most people find it hard to adjust to the ever changing prices of food. The elderly also find it difficult, so they economise by excluding foods which seem too expensive and reducing the amount they eat of foods they consider essential. *Tactful help* in budgeting and an explanation that food is an essential, not a luxury, can help to overcome these problems.

Therapeutic diets. Dietitians do not always realise that some therapeutic diets cause malnutrition in the elderly, for example:

1. Keeping to a strict weight reduction diet long after the ideal (target) weight has been reached
2. Self-imposed exclusion of carbohydrate in a well-intentioned attempt to control diabetes.

The elderly who are prescribed special diets should see a dietitian regularly to check that they are still eating a nourishing balanced diet.

Teeth. Healthy teeth and gums are essential for comfortable eating and effective chewing. The daily energy intake of the elderly people with ill-fitting dentures is 200–300 kcal less than for those with adequate dentition. This is because eating is uncomfortable and these people gradually adopt a soft bland diet. Poor chewing of food is sometimes the cause of indigestion.

Prevention of malnutrition

Malnutrition could be prevented if all the people who care for the elderly were aware of the risks and the contributory factors. Health education programmes aimed at the elderly, pre-retirement groups and those who work with the elderly are of great value.

Pre-retirement courses. These courses are run by local authorities and by some firms for those employees who are approaching retirement age. These courses should include several sessions in which nutrition is discussed, and should include a demonstration of easy cooking methods and ideas for menu planning for one. The following are topics which should be included in the nutrition sessions of a pre-retirement course:

1. Basic good nutrition

1g alcohol - 7 Kcal.

2. Meal planning
3. Encouragement of men to cook
4. Stimulation of an interest in food and cooking
5. Prevention of obesity
6. Importance of fibre in the diet
7. Importance of good dentition
8. Emergency food store
9. Value of convenience foods.

The emergency food store. There are times when because of illness or bad weather the elderly are unable to go shopping. To ensure that this does not mean that they have nothing to eat, they should keep a store cupboard. Some suggestions for such an emergency store include:

Tinned soup
Dried fruit
Long life milk
Tinned fish
Instant mashed potato
Instant fruit juices
Breakfast cereals
Tinned meat
Crispbread or biscuits

Nutrition education

Even the frail 75+ age group can benefit from nutrition education. This is based on a few simple dietary changes which will improve their diet (Table 14.3).

Table 14.3 Simple changes to improve the diet of the elderly

1. Have a glass of fruit juice every day
2. Have a fortified wholegrain cereal (e.g. Weetabix) with milk for breakfast
3. Try to eat meat or fish once every day
4. Have a milk drink at bedtime
5. Eat at least one serving of vegetables every day.

Home helps

These give invaluable support to the frail and housebound elderly. They frequently do the shopping as well as preparing the only cooked meal of the day. Home help organisers often hold nutrition seminars for their staff to ensure that home helps are aware of the potential risk of malnutrition in the elderly.

Meals on Wheels

Only 2½–3 per cent of the elderly population receive these. The number of meals each individual receives in a week depends both on the individual's infirmity and the local resources. Although this service has been running for many years there are some problems associated with it.

Portability. Not all meals travel well: some arrive at their destination tepid and unappetising.

Loss of nutrients. The nutritional value of a meal which is served and kept warm deteriorates. A survey carried out in Reading showed that after the meal had been kept warm for an hour, it had lost half of its vitamin C content and half of its thiamin content. Another survey has shown that for some recipients of Meals on Wheels, their diet contains less vitamin C on the day that the meal is provided than on the days when they cater for themselves!

Punctuality. It is impossible to provide all recipients of meals with a lunch at 12.45 pm. The elderly have created their own routine and often become set in their ways, so they do not like their lunch to arrive at 11.15 am or 1.45 pm.

Food will only improve nutritional status if it is eaten. The meal which is shared with the cat, or half kept for tomorrow will obviously not be so beneficial. The contribution of the social contact of the meal being delivered is important. When new methods of improving this service are being considered. this must be taken into account as well as the nutritional value of the food.

Lunch clubs

If transport is available, this is the ideal service. The meal does not have to travel, so a wider variety of dishes can be served and there is less deterioration of the vitamin content. The club also provides social contact and a pleasant dining environment.

Institutional catering for the elderly

All residents, whether in a long-stay geriatric ward, or local authority home, should look forward to and enjoy their meals. This can be accomplished by careful menu planning. Residents should be involved in this and if possible a menu card should be available beforehand showing the choice of dishes. Pureed meals must only be served as a last resort as they look unappetising and if the senses of taste and smell have deteriorated, they will all taste the same.

Carefully laid tables. As many people as are able should eat at a table which is attractively laid. Those who are able should pour their own tea, serve their own vegetables, etc.

Time. Time should be allowed for the meal to be eaten in a relaxed, leisurely manner.

Portion size. Serve small attractive portions with second helpings available and offered.

CONCLUSION

Everybody has to eat. Food is the most important part of the life of some old people and meal times the most important part of the day. It should be a source of health and pleasure to them all.

QUESTIONS

1. Which nutrients are likely to be low in the diet of an elderly widower?
2. Why is sunshine important in the elderly?
3. Suggest a nutritionally adequate meal, made from convenience foods that would be suitable for a single elderly lady.
4. Give three simple rules that could be implemented to improve the nutritional status of the elderly.
5. How would you make meal times on a geriatric ward more pleasant for your patients?

15

The nutritional problems of ethnic minorities

SUMMARY

1. It is important that all hospital patients receive a diet which is both acceptable and nutritionally adequate.
2. Many religions have strict dietary laws which must be obeyed.
3. It is necessary to understand these laws so that suitable meals can be offered and the appropriate dietary advice given.
4. Immigrants who find it difficult to obtain their traditional foods in sufficient quantities can develop nutritional deficiencies.
5. Nutrition education is very important in preventing these deficiencies in immigrants especially those from India and Pakistan.

INTRODUCTION

Towns and cities in this country are cosmopolitan centres with residents from all over the world. Immigrants come from India, Pakistan, the West Indies, Europe, Ireland, Australia and Canada. All bring with them their own traditions and cultures.

140

It is usual for immigrants to settle in the same area as their relatives and friends, who can help them to find work, accommodation and adjust to the new culture. Immigrant communities develop which retain much of the immigrants' original culture. An important part of any culture is food, whether it is the 'fast food' of North America or the curry of India. Food choice is governed by food availability, personal preference, tradition and upbringing and, for some people, by religious laws. Religious food laws developed for a variety of moral and practical reasons which include an abhorrence of slaughter, hygiene and a method of giving a group its own identity.

When unwell and in the strange surroundings of a hospital everybody likes to eat familiar food. The immigrant population is no exception. It is not usually possible to provide them with their traditional diet but if nurses understand which particular nutritional deficiencies are likely to occur and why certain foods are forbidden, they are able to ensure that whilst in hospital immigrant patients receive a diet that is nutritionally adequate and does not offend their religious beliefs. People from all over the world are resident in this country and nutritional disorders are not restricted to any section of this population. Their choice of food is governed by availability and religious laws. This chapter describes the dietary laws of the major religious and social groups of the world.

ASIAN IMMIGRANTS

Immigrants from India, Pakistan, Bangladesh and Indians from East Africa are grouped together as Asian immigrants. Their particular dietary problems are well understood. The traditional diet is based on cereals and vegetables. It is wrong to assume that all immigrants from the vast Indian sub-continent have the same diet. There are many regional variations. These are due to differences in religion, climate and tradition.

Climate

The diet is based on locally produced foods and the type of food grown depends on the local climate.

N.W. India and Pakistan have a temperate climate. Wheat

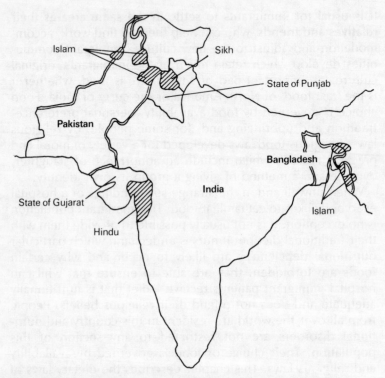

Figure 15.1 India, Pakistan and Bangladesh: showing areas from which Indians and Pakistanis have emigrated to the United Kingdom and the majority religion.

is grown as the staple cereal and is made into chapattis. These are flat cakes which are either cooked on a griddle or shallow fried and are eaten at every meal. Grazing is available for cows, so milk and milk products are included in the diet and ghee (clarified butter) is used for cooking. The vegetables grown include potatoes, carrots, cauliflowers and cucumbers.

Gujarat is an arid state. Millet is grown and ground into chapatti flour. Gujaratis in Britain use wheat chappati flour because it is easier to obtain and cheaper than millet flour. There is less grazing available for cows, so the diet contains less milk and yoghurt, and groundnut and mustard seed oils are used instead of ghee for cooking. The vegetables grown are members of the gourd family. Gujaratis are unfamiliar with most of the vegetables cheaply available in Britain.

Bangladesh. In the monsoon season much of this area which is a fertile alluvial plain is flooded. Rice is grown as the staple cereal and a lot of fish, both sea and fresh water, is eaten.

Asian religions

Most Asian immigrants adhere devoutly to their religions and the restrictions they impose. The three major religions are Islam, Hinduism and Sikhism. The dietary laws are summarised in Table 15.1

Hinduism

This is the historic faith of the entire sub-continent. Many of the Hindu beliefs and customs have been incorporated into the Islamic and Sikh religions. In Britain it is the immigrants from Gujarat and East Africa who are Hindu.

Hindu dietary laws
1. All life is sacred. No food that involves the taking of life can be eaten.
2. The cow is a sacred animal though milk and milk products can be eaten.

Fasting. Devout Hindus believe that fasting influences events, so they fast frequently, e.g., a woman will fast when her husband or child is ill. Fast days are decided on by the individual, after discussion with the priest, and are not predetermined. Hindus do not fast by abstaining from all food and drink but by restricting the amounts and types of foods they eat. Some people only eat foods that are considered pure on a fast day. These foods include fruit, nuts and potatoes.

Sikhism

This is a reformist sect of Hinduism which rejects the caste system. Even though Sikhs are one of the smallest religious groups in India, 80 per cent of Asian immigrants in Britain are Sikhs. Like Hindus the Sikhs believe that the cow is a sacred animal. Some Sikhs eat meat but none eat beef.

Islam

This is the religion of Muslims. Muslims come to Britain from Pakistan, Bangladesh, the Middle East, Malaysia and Africa. Muslims are forbidden to eat pork and pork products and must not drink alcohol. Although they are not vegetarian, any meat that they eat must have been killed in a special way. This is called Halal meat.

Ramadan is the ninth month of the Islamic (lunar) year. Muslims are expected to fast during the daylight hours of Ramadan. Everyone over the age of 12, except those who are ill, travelling, pregnant or breast feeding, is expected to fast. A person who is exempt from fasting during Ramadan is expected to make up the fast time at a later date. When Ramadan occurs in the summer, the period of fasting is much longer than if it falls in winter.

Ramadan dates	Start	Finish
1984	2 June	2/3 July
1985	22 May	20/21 June
1986	12 May	10/11 June
1987	2 May	31 May/1 June

It is not until the year 2000 that Ramadan occurs during the British winter.

Table 15.1 Summary of the foods eaten by the different religious groups of Asian immigrants

	Strict Hindus and Sikhs	Hindus	Sikhs	Muslims
Milk, yoghurt, ghee	yes	yes	yes	yes
Cheese	yes	yes	yes	yes
		(if it is not made with rennet)		
Eggs	no	rarely	sometimes	yes
Beef	no	no	no	Halal
Chicken	no	rarely	sometimes	Halal
Lamb	no	rarely	sometimes	Halal
Pork	no	no	rarely	no
Fish	no	no	yes	if it has fins and scales
Fruit	yes	yes	yes	yes
Vegetables	yes	yes	yes	yes
Pulses	yes	yes	yes	yes

Indian cooking methods and traditional foods

Many of the foods included in the Western diet are not excluded from the Asian diet because of religious reasons but because the flavour is unfamiliar or there is uncertainty about how it should be cooked. For example, it is customary here to serve plain boiled vegetables but this is never done in India. Vegetables are either fried or stewed with spices and meat or pulses. They are then served with chapatti and rice, or eaten raw in a salad dressed with lemon juice and spices. Over 100 spices are used in Indian cookery; different amounts of a variety of spices are added to each dish to give it its characteristic flavour. Indian patients find a hospital diet very bland. One way of overcoming this is for them to season their food with chilli powder or bottled chilli sauce instead of salt and pepper. Those immigrants who do eat meat are not used to eating it at every meal. Small amounts of meat are cooked with vegetables and served three or four times a week. Many Indians do not like the taste of texture of traditional British cheeses. The cheese that they are accustomed to is Paneer, which is a soft curd cheese with a mild flavour.

'Hot' and 'cold' foods

Foods are traditionally classified as 'hot' or 'cold'. Whether a food is hot or cold depends on religion, local and family tradition. In general, foods that taste sweet, bitter or sour are classified as cold and foods that taste salty or are high in animal protein are hot. Hot foods are believed to raise the body temperature and excite the emotions. Cold foods are thought to lower the body temperature, calm the emotions and make a person cheerful and strong. This food classification becomes important during illness, pregnancy and lactation, e.g., someone with a fever will eat 'cold' foods.

Nutritional deficiencies

A traditional Indian diet as eaten in India is nutritionally adequate. However, in some situations deficiencies of iron, folic acid, vitamin B_{12} and vitamin D occur.

Vitamin D (see ch. 6). There is a high incidence of rickets and osteomalacia amongst immigrants. It was assumed that this was due to diet and lack of sunshine. The diet is low in vitamin D and high in fibre and phytate which bind calcium making it unavailable. The traditional clothing and behaviour of the women and children prevents them from being exposed to sunshine. Recent surveys show that there is no definite cause for this deficiency but that it is probably due to a combination of environmental, genetic, cultural and dietary factors. However, increasing the dietary intake of vitamin D and increasing the amount of time spent in the sunshine are beneficial.

Foods rich in vitamin D which can be incorporated into Asian diets are margarine, evaporated milk, yoghurt and cottage cheese, which have been fortified with vitamin D, eggs and tinned oily fish.

Iron and B_{12} deficiencies. These can occur in any population where meat and animal products are not eaten. Iron rich foods which can be added to the diet are pulses, fortified breakfast cereals, oats, dried fruit and wholewheat products. Foods containing vitamin B_{12} are unboiled milk, dried milk, yoghurt and cottage cheese.

Folic acid deficiency. This occurs because the traditional vegetables are expensive, so smaller portions are eaten. Also, the less familiar British vegetables are overcooked and the folic acid is leached into the cooking water and thrown away. Folic acid rich foods are raw fruit and vegetables, green vegetables, dried fruit, nuts, wholewheat breakfast cereals and cheese.

In summary, the nutritional status of vegetarian immigrants is improved by more milk products, pulses, wholemeal products, fruit and vegetables, and that of non-vegetarians is improved by increasing the intake of these foods plus meat and eggs.

Weaning

Asian infants are usually weaned at an older age than their Caucasian counterparts. It is usual for them to be weaned onto the family food which has had some of the spices rinsed off. Many immigrant mothers now feed their children on commercially produced foods. They usually choose the sweet foods which ensures that the children do not receive any meat. This can cause problems as they develop a sweet tooth and do not become accustomed to the traditional spicy flavours. Community dietitians and health visitors give cookery demonstrations in Asian community centres and at English language classes. The aim of these classes is to improve the nutritional status of the entire family with particular emphasis on the use of suitable weaning foods, e.g., some of the family's meal mixed with baby rice.

Table 15.2 Sample hospital menus for Hindu, Sikh and Muslim patients

Hindu	Sikh	Muslim
Cereal and milk		
Toast and butter/margarine	as Hindu	as Hindu
Tea or milk		
Curried vegetables and pulses	as Hindu	as Hindu
Raw tomatoes and onion	or	or
Boiled rice	curried chicken	curried chicken
Rice with lentils		
Salad or Indian pickles	as Hindu	as Hindu
Yoghurt and fresh fruit		

The British expect their diet to have far more variety than Asians do. Asian meals are based on a pulse curry, rice or chapattis and relish or chutney. The tastes differ because of the numerous spice combinations used.

Judaism

Orthodox Jews are strict observers of their laws, ceremonies and traditions. They adhere to dietary laws (The Laws of Kashrut) as an act of self-discipline. These laws govern both the types of food eaten and its preparation, and are summarised below.

The laws of Kashrut

1. Meat must come from animals which chew the cud, are cloven hooved and have been killed ritually.
2. Milk or milk products must not be eaten at the same meal as meat. They must also be prepared and stored separately.

3. Fish must have fins and scales. Eels and shellfish are forbidden.
4. Jews should not cook or prepare food on the Sabbath.

The only nutritional disorder that Jewish immigrants are likely to suffer from is obesity. Jews are very good cooks; food and meal times are important parts of Jewish family life and tradition which may lead to over-indulgence. Most orthodox Jews live in well established Jewish communities where they are able to buy their meat from a Kosher butcher. The Jewish method of slaughtering animals for meat is very quick and ensures maximum blood loss. Once the animal has been killed, its carcase is salted and soaked in water. This process removes any remaining blood from the meat and is known as Koshering. In areas where Kosher meat is unavailable Jews will buy and eat Halal meat from Muslim butchers.

The only commonly eaten meat in a mixed diet which does not come from an animal that does not chew the cud is pork. The pig is considered unclean by Jews. Like the Muslims, Jews find pork and pork products repugnant. Hospitals can cater for the specific dietary needs of Jewish patients in two ways. The first is suitable for liberal Jews who, when in hospital, stop eating meat. In this way they can be certain that milk and meat are not eaten together and pork is not eaten. This is not suitable for some orthodox Jews so the second method is used whereby meals are either provided by relatives or frozen Kosher meals are bought and reheated in the hospital kitchen. The milk free margarine that is used by most Jews is called Tomor and is served in hospitals where there is a large Jewish population.

Jewish festivals

Passover. This is an eight day festival which occurs in Spring. Leavened bread cannot be eaten during Passover and it is replaced by unleavened bread which does not contain yeast.

Rosh Hashanah. This is a two day festival occurring in September. Many traditional foods, for example honey cake, are eaten during this festival.

Yom Kippur occurs in the Autumn and is accompanied by a 25 hour fast during which no food or drink is consumed.

Table 15.3 Sample hospital menu for a Jewish patient

Cereal with milk
Toast, butter and marmalade
Tea

Grilled fish with lemon
Mixed vegetables
Baked jacket potato
Fresh fruit

Cheese salad
Boiled potatoes
Milk pudding

West Indian immigrants

West Indians in this country are familiar with the foods available and their choice of food is not governed by any dietary or religious taboos. They are unlikely to suffer from nutritional deficiency disorders. Their use of oil for cooking most foods and fondness of sweet foods does in some situations lead to obesity and conditions which are associated with obesity, such as hypertension and diabetes. The Rastafarians are the one group of the West Indian population who are likely to be malnourished.

Rastafarianism. The popularity of this religion is increasing amongst young West Indians. Rastafarians believe that the Emperor Haile Selassie was their Messiah and that eventually all black people will return to Ethiopia, their promised land. Their dietary rules are a combination of the desire to eliminate all Western influences from their life and the Old Testament food laws. Strict Rastafarians are vegetarian and some are vegan (see Ch. 11). The less strict Rastafarians who eat meat, never eat pork. Foods that are prohibited include all canned, preserved and convenience foods and alcohol. Salt is not added when cooking. Foods that are acceptable are called Ital foods. These foods are unrefined cereals and organically grown vegetables. There has been very little research to investigate the nutritional status of this increasing group. It is likely that some of the young women and children will have a diet that contains insufficient supplies of iron, vitamin B_{12} and folic acid. The exclusion of animal products from the diet restricts the intake of B_{12} and iron. Few Rastafarians use

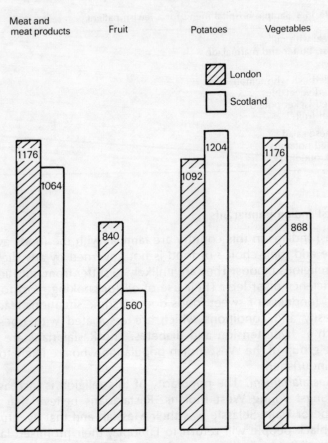

Figure 15.2 Comparison between the average weekly consumption of meat, fruit, potatoes and vegetables in Greater London and Scotland (in grams).

pulses frequently as a substitute for meat. Traditional Ital vegetables are expensive to buy. The vegetables that are eaten are usually cooked for a long time and the water, containing the folic acid, thrown away. Babies are not fed commercially produced foods: they are breast fed for a long time and weaned onto a high carbohydrate diet, based on cereals and starchy vegetables, which is not supplemented with the DHSS vitamin drops and does not contain any of the fortified baby foods.

This chapter describes the wide diversity of diets found among the residents of a large city. In addition to these, there are regional variations of the indigenous population. These are influenced by the region's geographical location, agriculture and traditions. For example, more fish is eaten in coastal areas and the Scottish eat less fruit and vegetables and more potatoes than the English. The differences between the average weekly intakes of meat, fruit, potatoes and vegetables in Greater London and Scotland are shown in Figure 15.2

QUESTIONS

1. What are the dietary differences between Hindus and Sikhs?
2. Which deficiency disorders are some Hindus likely to suffer from?
3. Why is this?
4. When do Jews fast?
5. Milk is a valuable source of many nutrients. When will Jews avoid it?
6. Name three protein rich foods which could be included in a vegetarian diet.

16

Diet in infancy, childhood and adolescence

SUMMARY

Good nutrition is essential for the normal development of children. Breast milk is the ideal food during the first months of life.

Dietary habits established during childhood are maintained for life. Infants should be weaned onto a varied and nutritious diet which encourages the development of healthy eating habits.

During the first few months of life the principal item of food is milk.

As the milk of each species is designed to meet the needs of the young of the species, breast milk is the food of choice for the human infant. Provided the mother's diet is satisfactory an infant fully breast fed will obtain from the milk, in an easily assimilated form, all the nutrients needed for the first four or five months.

A very substantial proportion of babies in Western communities are bottle fed. The reasons for this are complex and not fully understood. The mother herself may have an antipathy towards breast feeding, there may be insufficient privacy for her in the home, or she may be unable to breast feed if she goes out to work. Often insufficient encouragement is given at antenatal clinics and in hospital following delivery, where feeding practices may be designed to suit the hospital routine rather than the needs of the mother and the child. Sometimes breast feeding is not practicable because of illness of the mother or the child, or because the mother's milk secretion is inadequate for the infant's needs.

Feeding with modified cow's milk has been shown to be a satisfactory alternative provided it is correctly carried out. It can however in some circumstances present hazards to the baby. These are discussed in the section on artificial feeding. Nurses have a responsibility to give every encouragement to mothers who prefer, or who are prepared to breast feed. At the same time a sympathetic and balanced approach is called for. Those who cannot or who do not wish to breast feed should not be burdened with an unnecessary feeling of guilt which could in itself be harmful, but should be shown how to bottle feed successfully.

The Working Party on Infant Feeding of the Panel on Child Nutrition*, reporting in 1974, recommended that mothers should breast feed for the first four to six months of life, and in any case for a minimum of 2 weeks.

In underdeveloped and impoverished communities where the standard of education is low, bottle feeding is a major cause of infant mortality. Because of the expense of proprietary preparations, dilute mixtures are fed; also it is virtually impossible to prepare feeds which are bacteriologically safe. In these circumstances breast feeding can be essential to survival.

For the first three or four days after parturition the breasts secrete a small amount of a watery, yellow fluid of high protein content. This is known as colostrum. Milk secretion is not fully established until about the end of the first week.

Times of feeding

It is sometimes advocated that babies should be fed when they appear to be hungry rather than according to a set time-

* Committee on Medical Aspects of Food Policy.

table; this is known as demand feeding. On the other hand a feeding routine has obvious advantages for the mother and most babies will readily adopt such a routine. A feeding time-table however must be flexible, and the baby should not be made to wait for food if he is hungry.

Most infants adapt satisfactorily to a fourhourly schedule which allows for five feeds daily, at approximately 6 a.m., 10 a.m., 2 p.m., 6 p.m., and 10 p.m. In the case of very young infants, or those under 2.75 kg in weight, six feeds daily may be required, given at about 6 a.m., 9 a.m., 12 mid-day, 3 p.m., 6 p.m., 10 p.m. If the baby cries with hunger during the night an additional night feed is given. This can usually be discontinued after the first week or two.

Feeding routine

Emptying of the breasts is one of the strongest stimuli to milk secretion. As the baby may not take all of the milk from both breasts at each feed it is advisable to ensure that both breasts are regularly drained of milk by starting successive feeds with alternate breasts. In the initial stages when milk secretion is becoming established, it is advisable to express, either manually or by means of a breast pump, any milk remaining in the breasts at the end of the nursing period.

The baby will obtain most of the available milk from either breast in about five minutes. Ten minutes at each breast is therefore a sufficient allocation of time, and in some cases less will suffice. At the end of the feeding period the baby should be supported in a sitting position for ten to twenty minutes to permit the escape of air swallowed along with the milk. It may also be necessary to allow an interval for eructation of air during the course of the feed.

Adequacy of milk secretion

The supply of breast milk may be presumed to be adequate if the baby appears to be satisfied, sleeps for most of the time between feeds, and gains weight satisfactorily (see below). If the milk secretion is insufficient for the child's needs bottle feeds may be given immediately after the breast feeds. This is known as complementary feeding. Complementary feeds after the 6 p.m. and 10 p.m. breast feeds may be all that is required, and will help to ensure a good night's rest for both the mother and the child.

Vitamin supplements

These are discussed on page 160.

Expected body weight

When estimating expected weight it is customary to allow for some weight loss immediately after birth, which loss is usually made good by about the tenth day. A subsequent weight gain of 30 g per day until the end of the third month is then assumed. For example the expected weight of a 3-month-old infant, who weighed 3.4 kg (7 lb 8 oz) at birth, would be:

Birth weight + 30 grams per day with the exception of the first 10 days

$$= 3.4 \text{ kg} + (80 \text{ days} \times 30 \text{ g per day}),$$
$$= 3.4 + 2.4 \text{ kg},$$
$$= 5.8 \text{ kg} (12 \text{ lb } 12 \text{ oz}),$$

For the remainder of the first year a weight increase of 0.5 kg per month may be allowed for.

Variations from these figures are to expected. Babies do not gain weight at a constant rate. Many healthy babies show a more rapid weight gain than these figures indicate.

WEANING

Traditionally weaning is the term used to describe the change from breast feeding to a mixed diet, or to cow's milk given from a bottle. More recently it is taken as implying the introduction of mixed feeding.

Weaning from the breast should take place gradually. The disturbance to the baby is thus reduced to a minimum and the mother is less likely to suffer the discomfort of engorged breasts. One by one the breast feeds should be replaced by bottle feeds. Several days should be allowed to elapse after each replacement before another bottle feed is introduced.

If mixed feeding has already commenced it may be possible to give cow's milk from a cup, thus dispensing with the use of a bottle.

ARTIFICIAL FEEDING

Some comparisons between breast milk and cow's milk

Minerals. Cow's milk contains more calcium and phosphorus than human milk, and the ratio of phosphorus to calcium is greater. The high phosphorus content of cow's milk is a possible factor contributing to the low blood calcium level (hypocalcaemia) which is sometimes seen in the neonatal period, and which occasionally gives rise to tetany.

Cow's milk also contains more sodium and potassium than breast milk.

Protein. Cow's milk has a higher protein content than human milk. The proteins of human and cow's milk vary also in composition, the principal protein of human milk being lactalbumin while the principal protein of cow's milk is casein.

Fat. The fat of breast milk differs from that of butter fat in its fatty acid composition and is more readily absorbed, especialy by very young infants. The feeding of cow's milk, therefore, can result in incomplete utilisation of the energy value of the feed. Some manufacturers have attempted to simulate breast milk by using certain vegetable oils in their products. The effect of feeding dietary fats not found in breast milk on digestion and metabolism in the infant is not yet fully understood.

Some other considerations. Bottle feeding presents the opportunity to some mothers to over-feed the baby, either by careless measurement of the milk powder or pressing down a scoop not intended to be packed, or by using heaped scoops, or by adding extra scoops to a feed. There is also the temptation to add precooked cereal foods and rusks to the bottle feed instead of feeding them by spoon. The baby may be given another feed every time he cries when he may in fact be thirsty and requiring boiled water. Obesity is associated with much ill-health, in infancy as in adult life.

By feeding from the breast the mother is relieved of the responsibility of preparing feeds, with the attendant possibility of error, and as the milk is taken directly from the breast there is little opportunity for it to become contaminated with pathogenic bacteria. In the past gastroenteritis has been responsible for a high death rate among artificially fed infants. Although the incidence of gastroenteritis has declined greatly due to the production and sale of clean milk and the application of improved bottle feeding techniques, this disease still represents a hazard to bottle fed infants where standards of hygiene are poor.

Breast milk contains antibodies against certain micro-organisms, including *E. coli,* of which some strains are important in causing infantile diarrhoea. Also the faecal flora of breast fed infants differs from that of bottle fed infants resulting in a higher acidity in the former case. There is evidence that these factors may be important in helping the baby to resist infection.

It is said that suckling promotes a sense of security in the infant; nevertheless a baby who is handled with care and affection will enjoy a sense of security whether or not he is breast fed.

Types of milk used for artificial feeding

Milks used for artificial feeding fall into two categories:
1. Unmodified, pasteurised cow's milk, normally boiled in the home as an additional safeguard.
2. Proprietary milks. These are prepared from cow's milk, but modified so that a closer resemblance to human milk is achieved. They are sometimes referred to as low electrolyte milks as a reduction in electrolyte, or mineral content is an important feature of their composition.

Some details of the composition of breast milk and the milks referred to above are given in Table 16.1.

Choice of milk

The Working Party on Infant Feeding of the Panel on Child Nutrition, already referred to on page 153, recommended, among other things, that when breast feeding is impossible modified proprietary milks are the best substitute. They also recommended that artificial milks when reconstituted should approximate to the composition of breast milk as nearly as is practicable, and should contain a concentration of protein and certain electrolytes lower than that of cow's milk and nearer to that of breast milk.

The final decision rests with the mother, and it should not be forgotten that babies have successfully adapted to cow's milk for many years. It must be emphasised that it is not an adequate source of vitamins D and C, and those who decide to feed with cow's milk should give supplements of these vitamins.

A proprietary milk can be used for the first six months or so, after which time when the baby begins to drink from a cup, cow's milk can be gradually introduced.

Food requirements of healthy infants

Fluid. A figure of 150 ml per kg (2½ oz per lb) body weight daily may be taken as a guide to fluid requirements. Additional fluid may be required in hot climates or during hot summer weather.

Protein. A breast fed infant obtains approximately 2 to 2.5 g protein per kg body daily. Cow's milk and breast milk proteins are equally effective in supplying the amino acids needed by the infant. Nevertheless an intake of approximately 3 g cow's milk protein per kg body weight daily (1.5 g per lb) has been recommended.

Energy. An intake of approximately 110 kcal, or 460 kj per kg (50 kcal per lb) per day is recommended.

These criteria are met by any of the milks listed in Table 16.1, prepared for normal feeding according to the manufacturer's instructions. The figures given above are intended as a guide and should not be applied in an arbitrary manner when assessing the needs of individual babies.

An infant should be given as much of the milk food as he requires to satisfy his appetite. It should however always be reconstituted with the appropriate amount of water, and never given in a concentrated form.

Expected body weight

A means of estimating expected body weight is described on page 155.

Food preparation and administration

Before preparing a feed the hands should be washed thoroughly, using soap, hot water and a brush. Each feed may be prepared as required, alternatively feeds for 24 hours can be prepared in bulk, bottled, and refrigerated.

Mothers should be instructed to use the appropriate scoop provided with each milk powder, and in accordance with the manufacturer's instructions. A packed scoop may be required. More often the scoop should be lightly filled, not pressed down, but levelled off with the sharp edge of a knife. The mother must also understand that the scoop is meant for measuring the milk food only and should not be used for the water, which should be measured in a jug, or in the feeding bottle. Instructions for reconstituting a liquid milk requiring the addition of water should be followed with equal precision.

It is of the greatest importance that the mother should hold the baby in her arms during the feeding period so that he may enjoy the sense of security associated with breast feeding. At the same time she herself is able to give her attention to the details of technique described below. The practice of propping up the bottle in the cot or pram with the teat in the baby's mouth is dangerous, as milk may enter his lungs.

Before feeding the baby the milk mixture should be brought to the correct temperature by standing the bottle in a jug of water which may be either hot or cold, as required. The temperature of the milk should be tested by shaking a few drops out of the hole in the teat on to the back of the hand. It should feel slightly warm. The hole in the teat should be sufficiently large to allow the milk to drop out slowly when the bottle is inverted. The baby should be able to finish the feed in fifteen to twenty minutes. If the hole requires to be enlarged, this may be done with a red-hot darning needle.

It is important to ensure that the teat is filled with milk while the baby is feeding, otherwise a considerable amount of air will be swallowed. The teat should be removed from the baby's mouth at frequent intervals to permit air to enter the bottle. If the teat becomes collapsed during administration of the feed it should be gently eased away from the edge of the bottle opening so that air may enter. As with breast fed babies, time must be allowed for 'bringing up wind' both during and at the end of the feed.

Vitamin supplements

The vitamin content of human milk reflects the vitamin D status of the mother and the adequacy of her diet. If she is healthy and eating a good diet her baby will not require vitamin supplements. However if there is any doubt, and particularly in the case of immigrant Asian mothers whose diets may be deficient in vitamin D, and who may lack exposure to sunlight, the baby should be given the full dose of Welfare vitamin drops. Welfare vitamin tablets are provided for expectant and nursing mothers. These contain the vitamins A, C and D and the minerals calcium and iodine.

Proprietary milk powders sold for infant feeding are already fortified with vitamins A, D and C. Liquid cow's milk on the other hand is a poor source of both ascorbic acid and vitamin D, and further destruction of ascorbic acid results from storage and from heat treatment of the milk.

The vitamin drops provided at the Infant Welfare Clinics supply a satisfactory supplement of all three vitamins in a single dose and are suitable for both breast fed and bottle fed babies. They are available at minimal cost and are free of charge in approved cases. The dosage on the bottle should be followed carefully as excessive amounts of vitamin A and D can be harmful. Young children should be given them every day until they are two. Children between the ages of two and five should be given them during the winter months, October to the end of March.

Mixed feeding

By the fourth or fifth month an infant may be taking 200 ml or more of milk at each feed, and in order to provide for still-increasing dietary requirements it is necessary to enlarge the scope of the diet to include foods which will supply the necessary nourishment in a more concentrated form. Thus a mixed diet becomes necessary. Both breast milk and cow's milk are poor in iron content. An infant at birth has a store of iron which is sufficient for its needs for the first few months of life. To delay the introduction of mixed feeding beyond the fourth or fifth month may lead to the development of anaemia. Proprietary milks, however, such as those listed in Table 16.1, contain added iron.

The mother may be advised to give a pre-cooked cereal, such as Baby Rice, before the 10 a.m. feed. The cereal is mixed to a fluid consistency with some of the prepared milk mixture. A teaspoon should be used for feeding. The amount need not be restricted, but will vary with the age of the child. One or two teaspoonfuls will probably be adequate to begin with. If the baby appears at first to spit out the food this does not necessarily mean that he dislikes it, but may be due to the fact that he is not yet able to use his tongue to propel the food to the back of his mouth. As the baby becomes accustomed to taking food from a spoon a thicker mixture may be given.

Later, when the cereal is well accepted, one or two teaspoonfuls of sieved vegetable or tomato juice may be given before the mid-day feed. After some days another vegetable may be offered, and by stages the baby may be induced to accept, in addition to the vegetables, finely mashed potato moistened with plenty of gravy, stock or vegetable water, and shredded or minced meat, fish or offal. Foods must be sieved or finely minced as the baby is not able to chew, and not being accustomed to lumps, usually spits them out. The many proprietary foods may prove useful at this stage, particularly the dehydrated foods which can be reconstituted in small amounts. The proprietary foods often taste bland. Extra salt or sugar must not be added to enhance the flavour.

The next move is to introduce another spoon feed at 6 p.m. By degrees the diet is further extended. One or two teaspoons of egg yolk may be mixed with the cereal food, increasing by degrees to a whole egg. Other suitable foods include egg custard, milk and cereal puddings such as custard and corn-flour, porridge, sieved fruit, and finely grated cheese, which may be sprinkled over the cereal food or the potato.

Most infants take readily to mixed feeding. It is important, however, to avoid forcing foods which are not well accepted, and should the baby resist all efforts to give food other than from the breast or bottle the attempt should be abandoned and another trial made after a week or two.

As the infant's appetite for solid food increases he will take less milk from the breast or bottle. At the age of 5 or 6 months

Table 16.1 Composition of some milks

| Type of milk | g per 100 ml | | | Calories per 100 ml | mg per 100 ml | | | | |
	Protein	Fat	Carbohydrate		Iron	Sodium	Potassium	Calcium	Phosphorus
Cow's milk	3.4	3.7	4.8	66 (277 kj)	0.10		160	120	95
Breast milk	1.2	3.8	7.0	67 (281 kj)	0.15	15	55	33	15
Proprietary milks prepared for feeding									
SMA	1.5 cow's milk protein	3.6 a blend containing vegetable oils	7.2 lactose	65 (273 kj)	1.27	25	74	56	44
Cow and Gate V Formula	1.85 cow's milk protein	3.25 a blend of vegetable oils	7.2 lactose	65 (272 kj)	0.65	26	87	64	50
Cow and Gate Babymilk Plus	1.85 cow's milk protein	3.45 butterfat	7.1 lactose	65 (272 kj)	0.65	26	85	64	50
Ostermilk Complete Formula	1.7 cow's milk protein	2.6 butterfat	8.6 maltodextrin and lactose	65 (273 kj)	0.9	26	71	61	50
Improved Formula Ostermilk Two	1.77 cow's milk protein	2.45 butterfat	8.31 lactose and maltodextrin	62 (260 kj)	0.89	31	80	65	53

	Protein	Protein type	Fat	Fat type	Carbohydrate	Carbohydrate type	Energy					
Milumil	1.85	cow's milk protein	3.1	butterfat	8.4	lactose maltodextrin amylose	68 (286 kJ)	0.7	27	86	71	55
Cow and Gate Premium	1.80	casein/albumin ratio resembles human milk	3.45	a blend of vegetable oils & butterfat	6.9	lactose	65 (272 kJ)	0.65	22	60	48	31
SMA Gold Cap	1.5	casein/albumin ratio resembles human milk	3.6	a blend containing vegetable oils	7.2	lactose	65 (273 kJ)	1.27	15	56	44	33
Osterfeed	1.45	casein/albumin ratio resembles human milk	3.82	butterfat vegetable oils	6.97	lactose	68 (284 kJ)	0.96	19	57	36	31
Aptamil	1.5	casein/albumin ratio resembles human milk	3.6	butter and vegetable fats	7.2	lactose	65 (273 kJ)	0.7	18	98	57	35

he should be encouraged to take milk from a cup, and bottle or breast feeds may be gradually dispensed with. The 10 p.m. feed should be continued until the baby is sufficiently satisfied by the evening meal to sleep until morning.

After the appearance of teeth, rusks and biscuits should be given. By degrees meals begin to follow the adult pattern. The 10 a.m. feed becomes breakfast at about 8 a.m., the 2 p.m. feed becomes the mid-day meal, the 4 p.m. feed is dispensed with and the last meal of the day is given around 6 p.m. If the baby wakes early in the morning a drink of fruit juice may be given.

By the end of the first year the dietary regimen should be similar to that outlined on page 166. Young children like to copy their elders, and at the family table enjoy sharing what they see on mother's or father's plate. Thus an opportunity is provided to establish good eating habits by setting a good example.

THE TODDLER AND PRESCHOOL CHILD

At this stage the diet should follow the adult pattern. As the teeth develop the child should be encouraged to use them and should be given such foods as raw apples, chopped lettuce, and vegetable and other foods in less finely divided form. Quantities should be adjusted in accordance with appetite. Where the feeding of young children is concerned certain points require special mention.

1. The value of milk in the diet of the child has been demonstrated. Nevertheless it is not necessary, or even desirable, to encourage the consumption of milk in large quantities. An intake of 500 ml daily is sufficient. An excessive consumption of milk tends to blunt the appetite for other important foods. Emphasis should be on a varied diet, containing fruits and vegetables, meat, offal, fish, cheese and egg. If a wide range of food is introduced during the first year there is less likelihood of food refusal later.

2. It should be appreciated that appetite will vary from meal to meal and from day to day, and that a healthy child should not be forced to eat when he is not hungry. Sweets, biscuits

and similar titbits should not be over-indulged in, and the appetite should be permitted to regulate the quantity of food taken at meal times.

3. Food likes and dislikes should not be discussed in the child's hearing. A child enjoys occupying the centre of the stage, and when he discovers that food refusal makes him the object of adult interest and concern he is not slow to take advantage of the fact.

4. The best way of introducing a child, one year of age or younger, to a varied diet is to let him sit at the table for the family meals. He is then likely to want a share of what he sees everyone else having, especially if he has not been given too many between-meal snacks.

5. In infancy almost the sole dietary sources of vitamin D are the proprietary milks and pre-cooked cereal foods fortified with this vitamin. When these foods are discontinued, vitamin D intake can be extremely low. A vitamin D supplement should therefore be continued during the second year of life at least.

6. In childhood, when dietary habits are being established, dental hygiene requires consideration. The remains of sugary and starchy foods lodging between the teech provide a medium for the growth of bacteria which produce acids capable of eroding dental enamel (Ch. 17). Biscuits and sweets should not be eaten between meals.

SCHOOL CHILDREN AND ADOLESCENTS

During childhood and adolescence the dietary pattern is similar to that of adult life. It is important to ensure that the large appetites of young people are satisfied with substantial and well-balanced meals. An intake of 500 ml milk daily is desirable, and the inclusion of a wide variety of foods will help to ensure that the diet is adequate. Young people who have developed good dietary habits in their own homes will be likely to select wisely for themselves in school, university or works canteens, and in their turn pass on good habits to the next generation.

Menu suitable for a child aged one year

Breakfast (8 a.m. approx.)
Fruit juice.
Small serving (2 to 3 tablespoons) porridge or pre-cooked cereal with milk.
Small piece bread or toast with butter or margarine.
Breakfast savoury such as lightly cooked egg, chopped bacon or fish can be offered sometimes.

Mid-day meal (12 mid-day approx.)
1 to 2 tablespoons flaked fish, or meat finely chopped or minced, or finely grated cheese.
2 tablespoons mashed potato.
Vegetable finely mashed.
Gravy or vegetable water to moisten.
Milk and cereal pudding, or egg custard, with the addition of stewed fruit occasionally.
Milk to drink.

Evening meal (4.30 p.m. approx.)
Pre-cooked cereal food and milk, with grated cheese or ½ egg, or lightly cooked egg with thin bread and butter, or thin sandwiches of bread and butter with grated cheese, chopped bacon or other meat, sardines or egg. Mashed banana, stewed fruit or jelly. Milk to drink.

QUESTIONS

1. What advice would you give to a mother who is breast feeding, to help her maintain an adequate supply of milk?
2. What vitamins are provided by the vitamin drops issued by Welfare Foods Distribution Centres?
3. In what circumstances could a breast-feeding mother be advised to take them?
4. What suggestions would you give to a mother as to when and how to introduce mixed feeding?
5. If a mother of a one-year-old child enquired about the advisability of giving vitamin supplements, what advice would you give her?
6. What advice would be appropriate for the mother of a ten-year-old child?

17

Diet and dental disease

SUMMARY

1. Dental caries and periodontal disease cause discomfort and tooth loss in the majority of the population.
2. Diet is important in the development and prevention of dental disease.
3. The incidence of tooth decay increases with the sucrose content of the diet.
4. Inclusion of fluoride in the diet provides teeth with protection against dental disease.

INTRODUCTION

Healthy teeth and gums are part of good general health. They are essential for good nutrition, understandable speech and an attractive appearance. Surveys show that one third of five year olds have had toothache and one sixth have had at least one tooth extracted. Each year 20 000 dentists fill 30 million teeth and extract five million (four tons). This costs the Health Service over £400 million. These distressing statistics are made worse by the knowledge that dental caries, the most common disease in industrialised countries, is preventable.

Teeth

Man has two natural sets of teeth. The first is the milk teeth. There are 20 milk teeth, which erupt between the ages of 6 months and 2 years and by the age of 12 have all been replaced by a set of 32 permanent teeth. There are four types of permanent teeth. Each type has a characteristic shape which enables it to be used for a specific function. The front teeth are the incisors, next to them are the canines, then the premolars and lastly the molars.

Permanent teeth

Type of tooth	No. in mouth	Shape	Function
Incisor	8	Chisel edged	Act as scissors for biting food
Canine	4	Conical	Tear off food
Pre-molar	8 ⎫	Square, the chewing edge has cusps	Act as millstones, food is ground between the cusps
Molar	12 ⎭		

Tooth structure

All teeth have the same basic structure as shown in Figure 17.1. The part which projects above the gum is the crown; the part which is embedded in the jaw is the root.

Enamel. The entire crown is covered with enamel. Enamel is the hardest material in the body. Its complex, dense, crystalline structure contains the minerals calcium, phosphate and fluoride. The covering of enamel protects the biting and grinding surfaces of the tooth.

Dentine and cement. The structure of these two layers is similar. It is like dense bone without any blood vessels. The dentine layer is harder than the cement.

Pulp. This is the core which contains the blood vessels and the nerve.

Root. The root of the tooth is embedded in a socket in the jaw and fastened by the periodontal ligaments which link the cement to the bone.

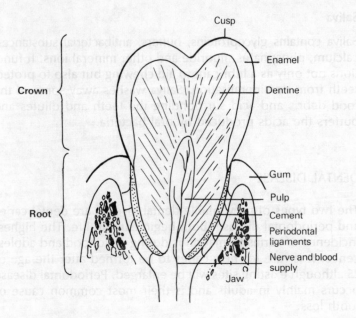

Figure 17.1 Cross-section of a molar tooth.

Tooth development

Permanent teeth take a along time to develop. They begin to develop at 32 weeks in utero and are complete by 9–12 years of age, even if not fully erupted.

Stages of development of adult teeth

32 weeks–3 years   At birth the jaws are already filled with developing teeth. The organic framework for enamel and dentine are deposited and calcification of the teeth starts.

3 years   The crown of the tooth is still buried in the jaw. It has reached its adult size but is not completely calcified.

6–7 years   Crown of tooth erupts into the oral cavity.

9–11 years   The development of the root of the tooth is completed.

Saliva

Saliva contains glycoproteins, buffers, antibacterial substances, calcium, phosphates, fluoride and other mineral ions. It functions not only as a lubricant to aid chewing but also to protect teeth from demineralisation. Saliva washes away some of the food debris and acid surrounding the teeth and dilutes and buffers the acids produced by oral bacteria.

DENTAL DISEASE

The two types of preventable dental disease are dental caries and periodontal disease. Both begin early in life. The highest incidence of caries formation is during childhood and adolescence. It is rare for new caries to be formed after the age of 25 although existing sites will be enlarged. Periodontal disease occurs mainly in adults and is their most common cause of tooth loss.

Dental caries

This is the progressive destruction of the enamel, dentine and cement of a tooth. In Medieval times it was thought that they were caused by worms in the teeth. It has been known since 1890 that caries only develop if three factors are present:
1. Susceptible teeth.
2. Substrate for cariogenic bacteria.
3. Cariogenic bacteria.
The ten steps of development of dental caries is illustrated in Figure 17.2.

1. Susceptible teeth. A tooth's susceptibility depends on nutrition during tooth development and on heredity. The availability of fluoride and good overall nutrition during the period of tooth development make it less susceptible. Genetically, the teeth of some people are more caries-resistant than those of others.

2. Substrate. Cariogenic bacteria metabolise carbohydrates as an energy source. Different bacteria are adapted to metabolise different carbohydrates. Sucrose, glucose and fructose are used, of which sucrose is the most important substrate.

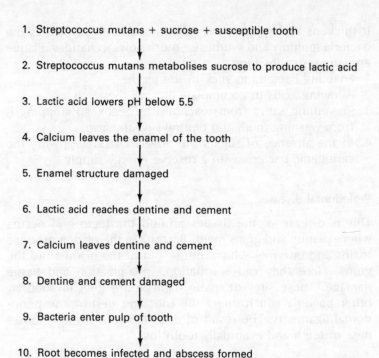

1. Streptococcus mutans + sucrose + susceptible tooth

2. Streptococcus mutans metabolises sucrose to produce lactic acid

3. Lactic acid lowers pH below 5.5

4. Calcium leaves the enamel of the tooth

5. Enamel structure damaged

6. Lactic acid reaches dentine and cement

7. Calcium leaves dentine and cement

8. Dentine and cement damaged

9. Bacteria enter pulp of tooth

10. Root becomes infected and abscess formed

Figure 17.2 The ten steps of development of dental caries.

3. Cariogenic bacteria. Certain strains of streptococci, lactobacilli and actinomyces are cariogenic. These bacteria metabolise carbohydrates to produce acids. *Streptococcus mutans* is the most important of the cariogenic bacteria. It metabolises sucrose to produce lactic acid which lowers the pH surrounding the teeth. Once the pH falls below 5.5 calcium ions start leaving the tooth enamel. This process is called demineralisation.

Dental plaque

This is the sticky whitish material that accumulates on the teeth. It consists of bacteria in a matrix of salts, proteins and polysaccharides. The polysaccharides are synthesised by the bacteria and act as a reserve substrate if sugar is not available. Plaque starts to form at the junction of the teeth and gums.

It thickens and spreads over the entire tooth surface as the bacteria multiply and synthesise more polysaccharides. Plaque encourages caries formation by:
1. Enabling bacteria to stick to the teeth.
2. Allowing acids to accumulate around the teeth.
3. Preventing saliva from reaching the teeth, so stopping it from washing them and neutralising the acid.
4. In the absence of sugars the polysaccharides provide the cariogenic bacteria with a reserve energy supply.

Periodontal disease

This is disease of the tissues around the teeth and occurs where plaque and gums meet. Bacteria in the plaque produce toxins and enzymes which diffuse out of the plaque into the gums. Here they cause irritation, inflammation and tissue damage. These sites of tissue damage are then invaded by other bacteria which infect the root and destroy the periodontal ligaments. The result of destruction of these is looseness of teeth and eventually tooth loss.

DIET AND DENTAL DISEASE

Nutrition and tooth development

Teeth start to develop before birth. At this stage the mother's general nutrition is important. There is no evidence to show that a diet high in calcium and vitamin D improves the strength of the developing teeth. However, the teeth of children of mothers who were poorly nourished in pregnancy are less resistant to caries formation later. Certain drugs taken during pregnancy will affect the calcification process of the tooth causing the enamel to be pitted and discoloured. This will only be noticed years later when the permanent teeth have erupted. The calcification of the tooth is a long process occurring over many years. If dietary fluoride is available it is incorporated into the enamel. The healthiest teeth develop when adequate supplies of all nutrients are available. However, two vitamins are particularly important. Vitamin A is needed for enamel development and vitamin D for dentine formation. Once the teeth are fully formed, vitamin deficiencies which cause gum damage, i.e. lack of vitamin C, will cause tooth loss.

Fluoride and tooth development.

The World Health Organization lists fluoride as an essential nutrient because of its importance in the prevention of caries development. The results of one survey conducted in Balsall Heath, to monitor the effect of the fluoridation of the water supply, showed that before fluoridation 8.7 per cent of 5 year olds had no caries and that four years later after fluoridation this percentage had increased fivefold to 47.7 per cent. In another study, addition of fluoride to the water reduced the incidence of caries on the smooth sides of teeth by 80 per cent. If fluoride is available for the entire period of tooth development and maturation it will provide the tooth with life-long protection. When fluoride is incorporated into the tooth the enamel is strengthened and made more resistant to demineralisation. The shape of the tooth is also changed. It is smaller and has fewer fissures. This is important because it is in these fissures that plaque and food debris can collect.

Fluoride in the diet

Water and soil contain fluoride in small and varied amounts. This means that most foods contain some fluoride but the amount will be very variable. The fluoridation of the water supply to a level of one part per million is the most effective way of ensuring that the diet contains a supply of fluoride that is both adequate and continuous. When the water supply is not fluoridated, fluoride tablets can be taken. However, there is the risk of overdosage. Excess fluoride causes the enamel of the permanent teeth to have a mottled appearance. Fluoride-containing toothpastes have a beneficial effect, but this is not as great as fluoride in the water or fluoride tablets.

Diet and dental caries

Aristotle was one of the first to link carbohydrates with tooth decay. He noted that the sugar in figs caused teeth to rot. A normal diet contains a variety of carbohydrate-containing foods but not all of them are cariogenic. The cariogenicity of a food depends on:

1. The physical form of the food
2. Type of carbohydrate in the food
3. Frequency of consumption of the food.

1. Physical form

Sticky foods that adhere to the tooth surface and become stuck between the teeth are the worst. This is because the bacteria are able to metabolise them for longer resulting in a prolonged period of low pH, so allowing longer for demineralisation of teeth. Hard, fibrous foods require a lot of chewing which is beneficial for teeth and gums. Chewing stimulates the flow of saliva which washes the teeth and dilutes and buffers any acids present. Fibrous foods have a slight abrasive effect and do not adhere to teeth. It used to be thought that finishing a meal with a fibrous food such as an apple or celery would clean the teeth. This is not true, since only superficial food particles are removed. However, these foods are still valuable as sugar-free snack foods.

2. Type of carbohydrate

Complex carbohydrates (starches) are large molecules. Large molecules cannot diffuse into the plaque so they cannot be metabolised by bacteria in the plaque. Smaller molecules such as sucrose, glucose and fructose diffuse freely.

Sucrose in the diet is without doubt the major cause of dental caries. It is the sugar most commonly eaten and is rapidly metabolised to produce acids. Sweets and the addition of sugar to drinks are not the only sources of sucrose in the diet. Sucrose is contained in many manufactured foods. Epidemiological evidence links increasing sugar consumption with increased caries incidence in many countries. In the U.K., caries incidence increased with the availability of sucrose in the nineteenth century. Wartime periods of sugar rationing have been accompanied by a reduction in the incidence of caries.

The acidity of some fruits can cause demineralisation when sucked and will lead to eventual destruction of the front teeth.

This is a particular problem if grapefruit and lemons are sucked, a habit common in Asian communities.

3. Frequency of intake

The mouth pH drops 2.5 minutes after eating a sucrose-containing food and stays low for up to an hour. This means that if sucrose is consumed three times a day, pH will remain below 5.5 for about three hours. The demineralisation which occurs during this time is sufficient to destroy the enamel progressively. If low concentrations of sucrose are consumed infrequently the demineralisation is slight and once the pH has returned to normal, remineralisation will occur.

Site of dental caries. This can be used to identify the probable food which caused the caries.

Caries site	Type of food
Front teeth	Sweet drinks in infant feeders
Smooth surfaces of teeth near gums	Boiled sweets
Between the teeth, particularly the molars and premolars	Biscuits, cakes and toffees

Sick children

Special attention must be paid to preventing dental decay in sick and handicapped children. This is because it is difficult to provide these children with dental treatment. Both dental procedures which cause the gums to bleed and those which require a general anaesthetic are potentially more hazardous for sick children.

Handicapped children are particularly difficult for dentists to treat.

Children in hospital are at greater risk of developing dental caries because they usually have free access to sugar-containing drinks and sweets. It is easy to understand how this arises but if this continues for a long time or new habits developed in hospital are continued at home, tooth damage occurs.

Another reason why sick children are more likely to develop caries is the addition of sugar to children's medicines in an attempt to make them more palatable. This is a particular problem if they are taken between meals and last thing at night over a long period of time. If the child is confined to bed, dental hygiene often suffers and when the medical condition or treatment causes a dry mouth, saliva will not wash the teeth or buffer the acids produced.

PREVENTION OF DENTAL CARIES

There are four important factors:
1. Incorporation of fluoride to strengthen teeth.
2. Efficient tooth brushing to remove plaque.
3. Dietary changes.
4. Regular dental treatment.

DIETARY CHANGES

The overall aims of the changes are to reduce both the amount and frequency of sucrose consumption.
1. Always choose the sugar-free alternative if one is available, e.g. puffed wheat instead of sugar puffs; cream crackers instead of custard creams.
2. Do not add sugar to drinks.
3. Do not add extra sugar to infant and baby foods.
4. Eat fruit, nuts, crisps, plain biscuits, cheese and raw vegetables between meal snacks instead of sweets.
5. Avoid sticky foods.
6. If sugary foods and sweets are eaten, they should be eaten as part of or at the end of a meal.

The food and pharmaceutical industries could also reduce the incidence of caries by making the following changes:
1. Stop adding sugars to infant and baby foods, fruit juices, vitamin preparations and paediatric medicines.
2. Reducing the amount of sugar added to manufactured goods.
3. Producing more savoury, sugar-free snack foods.

QUESTIONS

1. How can dental disease be prevented?
2. Which dietary factors are important in the development of dental caries?

18

The development of the science of nutrition; nutrition at national and international levels; malnutrition today

SUMMARY

The influence of nutrition on health has always interested man. The nutritional research of the last two hundred years concentrated on the identification and isolation of specific nutrients and their deficiency disorders. There is still much to be learned about the results of nutritional excesses and the relationships between diet and disease.

Man has always been intensely interested in food. It is only recently, however, that he has come to acquire a fairly precise knowledge of its nature and functions, which was made possible by application of advances in the sciences of chemistry and physiology which were not to take place until the eighteenth century and later. Nevertheless, although scientific knowledge was lacking, some valuable observations were made. Thus liver, now known to be an excellent source of vitamin A, has been recommended as a cure for eye diseases since ancient times, the earliest known references appearing in Egyptian writings. Certain herbs and fruits were among the remedies suggested for scurvy, and many seamen, including

178

Captain Cook, found the eating of fresh vegetables and fruits to be a cure for this condition. Fish liver oil had been used as remedy for rickets and painful limbs long before the discovery of vitamin D.

During the early half of the nineteenth century scientific methods were first applied to the study of nutrition, and foods were classified according to their nature and functions. Outstanding for their work in this field were the French scientist Lavoisier, who initiated the study of energy metabolism, and the German chemist Liebig, who made accurate analyses of foods, and studied also the functions of food in the body.

At the end of the nineteenth century the only known nutrients were carbohydrates, proteins, fats and certain inorganic elements. About this time, however, numerous experimenters—the most notable being Hopkins, whose work was published in 1912—showed that diets consisting of these substances in a purified form failed to support life, and that foods must also contain certain other nutrients which had not yet been identified.

Around 1896 Eijkman, a Dutch physician working in the East Indies, discovered that fowls fed on polished rice developed symptoms similar to those of beriberi, but were cured when unmilled rice was given. This observation led eventually to the realisation that rice polishings contained a dietary factor, lack of which was the cause of beriberi. In 1913 the American workers Osborne and Mendel, and McCollum and Davis, demonstrated the existence of an essential nutrient which was present in certain fats. There thus appeared to be two accessory food factors, very small amounts of which were needed in the diet. They became known as fat-soluble A and water-soluble B. The name 'vitamine' was suggested by Funk, who also put forward the suggestion that there were numerous 'vitamines', and that a deficiency of any one of these resulted in the development of a specific disease. This proved to be the case. The name proposed by Funk was adopted, with the terminal 'e' omitted after it had been shown that Funk had been incorrect in assigning these substances to the group known as amines.

Meanwhile investigations had been proceeding in other directions. It was shown that proteins differed in nutritive value, depending upon their constituent amino acids. The nutritional significance of the trace elements was recognised.

It is not proposed to enumerate here those who have been the principal contributors of the knowledge we possess to-day. It is hoped, however, that what has been said will bring it home to the nurse that the science of nutrition is in its infancy, and enable her to appreciate the advances which have been made in this comparatively short space of time. Many further problems await elucidation. Thus, while in the light of present knowledge it is possible to avoid the nutritional errors which result in deficiency diseases such as rickets and scurvy, not enough is known about the nature of the diet which will result in the greatest benefit to health—the optimum diet. An understanding of the nature of the metabolic processes has made it clear that certain errors in metabolism can result in disease in spite of the diet being adequate, and has shown the need for further studies in this branch of nutrition research. It is to be hoped that before long present investigations will throw more light on these and other problems confronting us to-day.

NUTRITION AT NATIONAL LEVEL

Public health administration as we know it, and of which food administration is a part, had its beginnings in the nineteenth century. At this time measures were urgently required to combat the evils resulting from industrialisation and consequent rapid growth of large towns, and legislation dealt with such matters as the employment of child labour in factories, sanitation, housing and local government. The Food and Drugs Act of 1860 (amended in 1872) dealt with food adulteration. In 1906 the Education (Provision of Meals) Act helped to provide for the needs of destitute children, and in the same year was held the first National Conference on Infant Mortality. In 1913 the Medical Research Committee (later to become the Medical Research Council) was appointed and plans were prepared for a study of rickets.

The outcome of the First World War (1914–1918) was influenced very considerably by the abilities of the warring nations to maintain food supplies. Advances in science had made it possible to assess nutritional requirements with some degree of accuracy, and the Government received much advice from scientific experts. This advice, although not always appreciated at the time, proved to be sound. In the United Kingdom a Ministry of Food was established. Although rationing was required there was no hunger or obvious evidence of malnutrition. In Germany, however, and in other European countries, widespread hunger occurred, and there was a striking increase in the incidence of rickets and other diseases. In the United Kingdom food restrictions had come to an end by 1921 and the Ministry of Food was dissolved in that year.

The interval between the two world wars included a period of industrial depression. At this time there was much scientific research into nutritional problems and the technicalities of food production and preservation. The importance of vitamins, minerals and proteins, especially in the diets of mothers and children, received widespread recognition. Dietary surveys were undertaken in order to ascertain how food consumption compared with estimated requirements. These investigations showed that many people were unable to purchase an adequate diet, and it become apparent that poor diets were the cause of much physical disability. In 1931 an Advisory Committee on Nutrition was appointed. In 1934 milk was made available at a subsidised price to all children attending public elementary schools.

When the Second World War broke out in 1939 much evidence was available on the nutritional status of the community and on the steps which would be needed to safeguard this important aspect of National Defence. A Ministry of Food was once more established. Steps taken to protect and improve the national diet included the institution of a rationing system, the economical use of shipping space and an increased home production of foodstuffs, the addition of calcium to flour and an increase in extraction rate, and the addition of vitamins A and D to margarine. Certain sections of the community were given priority in the allocation of food. For example the School Meals Service and the Milk in Schools Scheme were further developed, and there were additional allowances and vitamin A and D tablets for pregnant and nursing women, infants and young children. The public were taught, by means of posters, leaflets and demonstrations, how to make the best use of available foods. That the health of the populace as a whole improved in spite of the strain imposed by the war may be largely attributed to the steps taken to ensure that food was available for all sections of the community in accordance with their needs.

Many of the measures put into effect during the war were of a temporary nature. Others form a part of the structure of food administration at the present time.

Nutrition at national level to-day

At the present time legislation safeguards many aspects of the national diet. Much of this legislation is embodied in the Food and Drugs Act of 1955.

Composition of foods. In some instances food must conform to certain standards of composition. For example flour must contain specified minimum amounts of thiamin, nicotinic acid and iron to compensate for loss of these nutrients during milling. Most flour is also subject to the addition of calcium carbonate. Vitamins A and D must be added to margarine. Food standards relate also to the use of preservatives and colouring matter, and deal with food contamination. Foods other than those already mentioned for which standards of composition are laid down include ice cream, cream, fish and meat pastes, soft drinks and many others.

Labelling and advertisement of foods. Legislation forbids the false labelling or advertisement of food.

Food hygiene. The conditions under which food is prepared and distributed must conform to certain specifications.

Advisory bodies

On matters relating to the health of the community the Government requires the advice of scientific experts. Important advisory bodies where food and nutrition are concerned are the Food Standards Committee, the Medical Research Council, the Chief Medical Officer's Committee on Medical and Nutritional Aspects of Food Policy, and the Department of Scientific and Industrial Research. Of great importance also is the research work which is carried out in universities and in research units throughout the country.

Evidence of nutritional status

The Ministry of Agriculture, Fisheries and Food published annually details of total food, both home-produced and imported, which is available commercially in this country. The Ministry also published anually the result of the National Food Survey. This is a record from a sample of households of the amount of food purchased for home consumption, allowance being made for food grown at home, also meals taken elsewhere.

This information can be utilised to help pin-point at-risk groups and also to indicate national trends in food consumption.

Statistics such as those relating to maternal and infant mortality and heights and weights of children provide useful evidence of the health and nutritional status of sections of the community.

Education

Nutrition is only one of many factors intimately connected with the health of the community, which is related also to such matters as housing, sanitation, personal hygiene, immunisation and the control of infectious diseases. Progress in these numerous fields is to a great extent dependent upon effective health education. In this local authorities play an important part. Use is made of posters, leaflets and films, and information is disseminated through such media as ante-natal and infant welfare centres, schools, clubs and adult associations such as Women's Institutes. The Central Council for Health Education gives advice and provides teaching aids and training courses. Many radio and television programmes and well-informed articles in newspapers and journals make a valuable contribution to health education. Persons such as doctors, nurses and teachers, who have influence in the community, are of great value as health educators.

Community dietitians are employed by most Health Authorities. By promoting an awareness of the importance of good nutrition they hope to improve the health of, and prevent disease in, the local population. The community dietitian works with the Health Education Service, Health Care Team, local community groups, Social Services and the Education service, providing them with accurate nutritional information and helping them to implement this.

NUTRITION AT INTERNATIONAL LEVEL

We who live in a country where food is plentiful ought never to forget that in many parts of the world people are either constantly hungry, or do not get a balanced diet adequate for the maintenance of health.

This problem is not by any means new in the history of the human race, but has acquired a fresh urgency in modern times as a result of the rapid increase in world population which is taking place, and which is especially marked in regions such as India and the Far East where standards of nutrition are already inadequate. The matter is also one of great political significance. It is widely recognised that international security will remain unattainable while in many countries throughout the world people are not adequately fed.

International co-operation is essential if this problem is to be dealt with effectively. Machinery for dealing with food problems on an international basis is to be found in the United Nations, the agencies concerned in this work being the World Health Organization (WHO), the Food and Agriculture Organization (FAO) and the United Nations Children's Fund (UNICEF). These organisations are composed of representatives of the governments of the participating countries and their funds consist of contributions from member states. Governments requiring assistance in carrying out programmes designed to increase food production and to combat ill-health may apply for technical and financial aid from these organisations.

WHO, as its name implies, is concerned with the promotion of health, and is active in many fields. Its undertakings have included the drawing up of international sanitary regulations and the investigation of disorders such as goitre, kwashiorkor and anaemia, which are the cause of widespread ill-health.

FAO deals principally with the technical aspects of

producing and distributing food. Its activities have included the promotion of improved methods of agriculture and pest control, the development of industries such as fishing and dairying which will result in improvements in regional diets, and the training of technical experts.

These two agencies work in close co-operation, their activities in the field of nutrition being co-ordinated by the Joint FAO/WHO Expert Committee on Nutrition. Many projects have been carried out by the joint efforts of FAO and WHO. The publications of these organisations include statistical information, and reports and recommendations relating to many economic and social problems.

When the United Nations International Children's Emergency Fund (UNICEF) was set up in 1946 its object was to bring assistance to children in the countries which had suffered most as a result of the war. In the field of nutrition this assistance took the form of contributing foods high in nutritive value for inclusion in a daily meal to be provided by the governments of the countries concerned. Foods provided included those high in protein, much use being made of skimmed milk powder, of which large quantities were readily available on the American market. This scheme, as well as providing emergency relief, demonstrated the value of child feeding programmes, and led to expansion of the dairy industry in many countries, in which UNICEF participated.

In its present form, as the United Nations Children's Fund, UNICEF is engaged in promoting the welfare of children throughout the world, and especially in developing countries. Stimulus is given to school-feeding programmes and the development of maternal and child welfare services. Through these and similar media food is distributed and nutrition education is given. UNICEF has supplied many countries with milk-processing equipment, and in regions where protein deficiency is prevalent is developing the use of locally available foods of high protein content. In carrying out its nutrition programmes UNICEF maintains close co-operation with FAO and WHO.

European economic community

A Scientific Committee for Food had been formed within the EEC, to advise on such matters as food composition, processing, the use of additives, and the problem of food contamination.

Malnutrition today

Protein-energy malnutrition

In Chapter 4 we have seen that protein-energy malnutrition, affecting children up to 5 years of age, is a serious problem in developing countries; there is a high incidence in parts of Africa, India, South East Asia, and Central and South America. The condition is associated with anaemia and vitamin deficiencies. It is impossible to compute how many children are suffering from protein-energy malnutrition but a rough estimate will indicate the extent of the problem—11 million children may be suffering from severe, and 76 million from moderate, forms of the disease. In those treated in hospital the mortality rate can be as high as 40 per cent while in the survivors growth is impaired, and possibly also mental development.

Xerophthalmia

This condition, which occurs principally in infants and young children, results from deficiency of vitamin A. The cornea of the eye is affected and may be become ulcerated, leading to blindness. Countries where the disease is prevalent include India, parts of South East Asia, Pakistan, and parts of Africa and the Middle East. In these countries xerophthalmia is a major cause of blindness.

Nutritional anaemia

Information is lacking on the incidence, in developing countries, of anaemia due to folate deficiency; in India it has been shown to be present in a considerable proportion of women attending ante-natal clinics.

Iron-deficiency anaemia is known to be widespread throughout the world, and is particularly prevalent in developing countries where it is sometimes associated with hookworm infestation. It also occurs in the more sophisticated communities, especially among the poorer sections of the population. Pregnant women and children between 6 and 18 months of age are particularly at risk.

Endemic goitre

Endemic goitre occurs in varying degrees in several of the developing countries where there are areas of iodine deficiency. A simple means of prevention is by the use of iodised salt.

Obesity

Obesity is a major nutritional disorder, affecting the affluent communities of the world, where it is associated with much ill-health. Unlike the other conditions discussed it results from overnutrition.

Other nutritional disorders such as rickets, scurvy, beri-beri and pellagra are still seen in some countries and in certain circumstances, but are not major health problems.

QUESTIONS

1. Why is it important to monitor the nutritional status of a nation?
2. How is it done in this country?
3. Which nutritional deficiencies are commonly encountered in developing countries?
4. How can they be prevented?

19

Food in illness

SUMMARY

An important part of patient care is an understanding of his nutritional needs: it contributes to both his recovery and well-being.

Most patients receive meals based on a normal diet. However, in certain circumstances specific dietary modification or special diets are necessary.

INTRODUCTION

It is essential that nurses notice how much food their patients eat. It is easy to overlook the patients who are either not bothering to, or who are unable to eat sufficient food. These patients must be identified quickly so that they can be given a suitable diet with any necessary supplements.

It is necessary for nurses to pay attention to the appearance of a meal as well as its nutrient content. Food is only of nutritional benefit when it is eaten. A patient with a poor appetite is more likely to eat a meal if it looks attractive and tempting. The following points should be considered:
1. Meals should be served at sensible times.

2. The hospital menu should be planned to provide acceptable, nutritionally adequate meals for the majority of patients.
3. All cutlery, plates and trays used must be clean.
4. Meals must be served carefully, not 'thrown' onto plates.
5. Patients with small appetites should be served small portions of food.
6. Where possible the likes and dislikes of patients should be considered.
7. Food should be easy to eat—no wrestling with tough meat or searching for fish bones.

Light diet

The term light diet is applied to a type of diet which provides adequate nourishment in non-bulky and easily eaten form. Small portions should be given at the main meals with snacks in between. The following should be avoided: fried foods, especially starchy foods such as bread and potatoes which absorb a lot of fat; foods with a high satiety value, such as pastry and steamed puddings. Food liable to cause flatulence should be given with due regard to the personal idiosyncrasies of the patient; these include vegetables of the cabbage family, turnip, leek, onion, cucumber and melon. Suitable foods include meat, fish, poultry, eggs, grated cheese, milk and milk dishes, cream, butter, margarine, preserves, white and brown breads, toast, plain cake, fruit juices, and most vegetables and fruits provided they can be adequately masticated.

The use of the selective menu in hospital catering enables the nurse to disseminate the principles of good nutrition in a practical way as she guides the patient in his choice. The patient may also learn how to adapt his meals to the requirements of a special diet.

On the following pages are reproduced a set of hospital menu cards for twenty-four hours ready to be filled in by the patient, with the assistance of the nurse or dietitian. On the original cards each item is marked with a code indicating its suitability for certain diets: low fat (LF), and reduction (R). The items suited to the reduction diet are normally the basis for the diabetic menu. The coding has been omitted here, the intention being that the nurse, as she studies the various dietary modifications, can return to these menus and fill in the code for herself.

Many hospitals now use coloured sticky labels to label meals that are sent to the ward from the diet kitchen. The colours used are:

Pink	—reducing diet
Red	—diabetic diet
Blue	—low protein diet
Dark orange	—high protein diet
Yellow	—low fat diet
Green	—low sodium diet
Pale green	—low residue diet

The prescription of borderline substances usually regarded as foods

Certain special foods are available for the treatment of specific diseases; for example gluten free flour and bread for the treatment of coeliac disease; low protein flour and bread for the management of renal failure; modified milk foods for the treatment of milk intolerance.

In circumstances such as these, preparations normally regarded as foods are sometimes classified as drugs, and may be prescribed by a general practitioner. For detailed and up-to-date information the appropriate Department of Health should be consulted.

QUESTIONS

From the printed menu card (Fig. 19.1) select meals for:
1. A high fibre diet.
2. A low fat diet.
3. A reducing diet.
4. A light diet.

ROYAL VICTORIA HOSPITAL

WEDNESDAY A   LUNCH

Name ....

Ward ....

TICK SIZE OF PORTION REQUIRED

Small ☐   Normal ☐   Large ☐

All Dishes suitable for ordinary Diets.
Symbols indicate Special Diets.

1 ☐	Scotch Broth	
2 ☐	Strained Scotch Broth	
3 ☐	Fish Cake and Tomato Sauce	
4 ☐	Roast Beef	
5 ☐	Minced Roast Beef	
6 ☐	Yorkshire Pudding	
7 ☐	Grated Cheese and Egg	
8 ☐	Salad	
9 ☐	Diet Salad	
10 ☐	Roast Potatoes	
11 ☐	Creamed Potatoes	
12 ☐	Boiled Potatoes	
13 ☐	Brussels Sprouts	
14 ☐	Turnip	
15 ☐	Rhubarb Tart	
16 ☐	Custard Sauce	
17 ☐	Semolina Pudding	
18 ☐	Dessert Pear	
19 ☐	Ice Cream	

Please indicate your choice by putting an X in the box provided to the left of
the dish chosen.

Above Menu subject to change due to factors beyond control of the Board.

Figure 19.1 Specimen menu cards

ROYAL VICTORIA HOSPITAL

WEDNESDAY A   SUPPER

Name ....

Ward ....

TICK SIZE OF PORTION REQUIRED

Small ☐   Normal ☐   Large ☐

All Dishes suitable for ordinary Diets.
Symbols indicate Special Diets.

1 ☐		Cream of Tomato Soup ....
2 ☐		Fried Haddock ....
3 ☐		Steamed Haddock ....
4 ☐		Egg Sauce ....
5 ☐		Cold Roast Pork ....
6 ☐		Salad ....
7 ☐		Diet Salad ....
OR		
8 ☐	4	Ham Sandwich ....
9 ☐	2	Ham Sandwich ....
10 ☐		Garden Peas ....
11 ☐		Cut Celery ....
12 ☐		White Bread ....
13 ☐		Wholemeal Bread ....
14 ☐		Butter ....
15 ☐		Jam ....
16 ☐		Caramel Cream ....
17 ☐		Low Calorie Fruit Salad ....
18 ☐		Rice Pudding ....
19 ☐		Vanilla Ice Cream ....

Please indicate your choice by putting an X in the box provided to the left of
the dish chosen.

Above Menu subject to change due to factors beyond control of the Board.

Figure 19.1 *(cont'd.)*

ROYAL VICTORIA HOSPITAL

THURSDAY A   BREAKFAST

Name ....

Ward ....

TICK SIZE OF PORTION REQUIRED

Small ☐   Normal ☐   Large ☐

All Dishes suitable for ordinary Diets.
Symbols indicate Special Diets.

1 ☐	Bran Flakes	....
2 ☐	All Bran	....
3 ☐	Rice Krispies	....
4 ☐	Porridge	....
5 ☐	Sieved Porridge	....
6 ☐	Grapefruit Juice	....
7 ☐	Scrambled Egg (Diets only)	....
8 ☐	White Toast Slice	....
9 ☐	White Bread Slice	....
10 ☐	Wholemeal Bread Slice	....
11 ☐	Butter	....
12 ☐	Marmalade	....

Please indicate your choice by putting an X in the box provided to the left of the dish chosen.

Above Menu subject to change due to factors beyond control of the Board.

20

Diet in obesity

SUMMARY

Obesity causes illness, unhappiness and discomfort to many people. It always develops when energy intake exceeds energy requirement. The most successful method of treating obesity is by sensible dieting which requires the dieter to be well motivated and patient. Many dieters become frustrasted and disillusioned with their slow progress and need encouragement and support as well as nutritional advice from those treating them.

INTRODUCTION

When the energy intake exceeds the energy requirement, obesity develops: see Figure 20.1. Any food not immediately required for energy production is converted to fat which accumulates in the body. Fat is not isolated in particular areas of the body, it is spread diffusely throughout the body. In women of average build, 18 per cent of their body weight is fat whereas in men, the percentage is lower at 16 per cent.

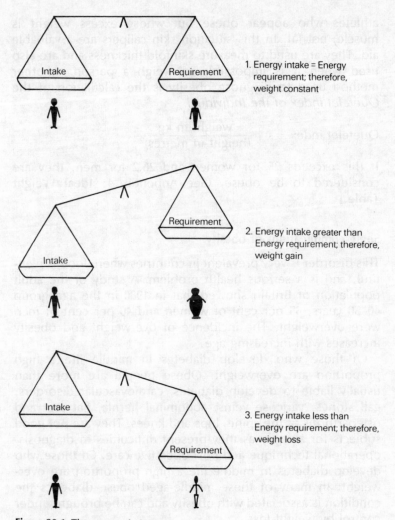

1. Energy intake = Energy requirement; therefore, weight constant

2. Energy intake greater than Energy requirement; therefore, weight gain

3. Energy intake less than Energy requirement; therefore, weight loss

Figure 20.1 The energy balance.

Diagnosis of obesity

In many situations, visual appearance is sufficient to indicate the presence of obesity. A person who is 110–120 per cent of his ideal weight is considered overweight and a person who weighs more than 120 per cent of his ideal weight is obese. There are occasions when this is not valid, for example, athletes who appear obese but whose excess weight is muscle, not fat. In this situation skin calipers are a valuable aid. They are used to measure skinfold thickness and are also used when it is impossible to weigh a person. Another method used to diagnose obesity is the calculation of the *Quetelet index of the Individual.*

$$\text{Quetelet index} = \frac{\text{weight in kg}}{(\text{height in metres})^2}$$

If this exceeds 25 for women and 26.2 for men, they are considered to be obese. (See Appendix 4: Ideal Weight Table.)

Some complications of obesity

This disorder is very prevalent in countries where food is plentiful, and is a serious health problem. A study of the adult population of Britain showed that in 1980 in the age group 40–50 years, 35 per cent of women and 40 per cent of men were overweight. The incidence of overweight and obesity increases with increasing age.

Of those who develop diabetes in middle life a high proportion are overweight. Obese people are more than usually liable to develop diabetes, cardiovascular disorders, gall stones, varicose veins, abdominal hernia, flat feet and osteoarthritis of the spine, hips and knees. They are not good subjects for surgery as they present difficulties in diagnosis, operational technique and post-operative care. Of those who develop diabetes in middle life a high proportion are overweight. In many of these middle-aged obese diabetics the condition is associated with obesity and can be brought under control by weight loss.

Causes of obesity

It has already been said that obese people eat more of the energy-producing foods than they require. Many factors play a part in bringing about this excessive food intake and thus contribute to the development of obesity (see Table 20.1).

There may have been a decrease in energy expenditure, perhaps following on a change of occupation, without a

Table 20.1 Some reasons for changes in energy requirements.

1. Change of job: for example, from working in a shop to sitting at a desk
2. Buying a car
3. Change of hobby: for example, from playing badminton to bowling

corresponding decrease in food intake. Some of the weight increase which occurs in middle life may be due to the fact that activity diminishes with age, whereas established food habits tend to remain unaltered. Eventually energy intake may be considerably in excess of expenditure.

Obesity also results from over-indulgence in cakes, chocolates and other confectionery, or starchy foods such as bread and biscuits. The establishment of good eating habits in childhood is a factor of great importance in the prevention of obesity.

Many people, especially women, find relief in eating during times of tension and unhappiness. In this case over-eating is part of the patient's adjustment to an unsatisfactory emotional environment, and food restriction without adequate management of the underlying emotional condition may result in mental disturbance (see Fig. 20.2). Women should avoid gaining an excessive amount of weight during pregnancy. Most women lose the fat gained during pregnancy. However, some who have always had to watch their weight use pregnancy as an excuse to give up controlling their weight. (Weight gain during pregnancy is discussed in Ch. 13.)

It has been suggested that the large appetites of some obese people may be due to factors affecting the satiety mechanism, which is controlled from centres at the base of the brain in the region of the hypothalamus. These factors, however, are not fully understood.

In some cases failure of equilibrium between energy intake and output may be the result of endocrine disturbance or genetic abnormalities, but most authorities believe this type of obesity to be relatively uncommon.

Attempts at present being made to ascertain if obese people metabolise food differently from the non-obese may eventually throw more light on the problem of obesity.

Prevention of obesity in infancy and childhood is a sensible

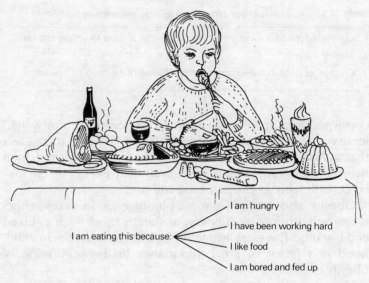

I am eating this because:
- I am hungry
- I have been working hard
- I like food
- I am bored and fed up

Figure 20.2

measure and a pattern of regular meal times should be established, without constant eating between meals. Unfortunately psychological factors can be difficult to resolve. For example parents who find themselves unable to give enough time and personal attention to their children may, without realising it, be compensating for this by overfeeding them. By the same token children who are emotionally deprived may get comfort from eating.

Fat

Unfair though it seems, some people can eat more than others without gaining weight even though they are of the same size and expend the same amount of energy. It has been suggested that this is related to the amount of brown fat in the body. Most of the adipose tissue of the body is white fat, where excess energy from ingested food is stored as fat. A small proportion of the body fat in localised areas is described as brown fat because of its appearance. This fat is metabolically much more active and is capable of burning off excess energy rapidly in the form of heat. Animals that hibernate and neonates have large amounts of brown fat, but most adults have a relatively small amount. Those who are prone to obesity have been reported to have less brown fat than lean people. In the lean person with more brown fat, any surplus energy consumed is metabolised rapidly by the brown fat and therefore not laid down as white fat stores.

Treatment

Whatever may be the underlying cause, the treatment of obesity necessitates a reduction in the energy value of the diet. An excess weight of 10 kg (1st 8 lb) represents an excess energy store of 80 000 kcal (336 MJ), or 266 Mars bars! It is obvious, therefore, that intake must be sufficiently restricted to make obese persons metabolise their own accumulated body fat in order to meet their energy requirements. Most people will lose weight if their energy intake is reduced by 2.1–4.2 MJ (500–1000 kcal). It is unfair to expect everbody to lose weight at the same rate on the same diet. The majority of moderately active people will lose weight on an allowance of approximately 4.2 MJ (1000 kcal) daily. For particularly active people with a normal energy expenditure of 12.6 MJ or more (3000 kcal) daily 8.4MJ (2000 kcal) may be a satisfactory allowance.

Exercise and weight reduction

Exercise increases energy expenditure, but does not contribute greatly to loss of weight unless it is regular and sustained. An hour's walk at 4 km (2½ miles) per hour on the part of a person weighing 70 kg (11st approx.) results in the expenditure of an additional 670 kJ (160 kcal) approximately, equivalent to 1½ slices (40 g) bread spread with butter. Exercise is of value along with dietary treatment but cannot replace it.

Table 20.2 Food consumption and exercise equivalents

Food portion	Energy content		Amount of exercise
7 squares milk chocolate	1.0 MJ	240 kcal	1½ hrs dancing
1 pint milk	1.6 MJ	370 kcal	1 hr swimming
1 packet potato crisps	0.6 MJ	150 kcal	1 hr cycling

Dietary management

The diet should conform as far as possible to the eating habits of the person concerned.

Reduction of the energy value of the diet is brought about by omitting sugar as such, and by restricting the intake of fat and foods high in starch.

It is important that adequate nutrition is maintained and a sufficient intake of protein, minerals and vitamins must be ensured. Bread and other flour products provide a substantial proportion of the iron of a normal diet. Thus when the energy allowance is reduced and the intake of these items is limited, foods with a high iron content should receive special emphasis; where possible liver should be taken at least once weekly.

Excessive hunger is avoided by the use of bulky and non-starchy vegetables such as cabbage, cauliflower, celery, lettuce, Brussels sprouts, tomato, marrow, carrot, turnip, and onion, and eating wholegrain and wholemeal products instead of the refined form. Sometimes it helps to begin the meal with a serving of unthickened soup, or to take some unsweetened tea or coffee, or a carbohydrate-free mineral between meals.

Rapid weight loss should be discouraged even though it is what every obese person wants. If weight loss is rapid, not only is fat metabolised but so is the lean tissue (muscle) and the glycogen stores of the muscle and liver are depleted. The rapid weight loss which occurs on short-term, very low energy diets is due to the metabolism of glycogen stores and the water and sodium diuresis that accompanies it. When energy intake is restored the glycogen stores are replaced and extra weight is gained.

Diet no. 1 (p. 202) will provide approximately 4.2 MJ (1000 kcal) daily and is particularly suited to persons for whom immediate weight loss is necessary. A weekly loss of from $\frac{3}{4}$ to $1\frac{1}{2}$ kg could be considered satisfactory.

Most people find it difficult to adhere to such a strict regimen and should be reassured that occasional breaking of the diet is natural, and should not cause undue despondency. An enthusiatic attitude on the part of the interviewer is of the greatest importance in securing co-operation.

The correction of obesity in the long term requires a permanent change of eating habits and this cannot be brought about overnight. For many it may be helpful to aim for a slow weight loss based on a gradual, and hopefully permanent, change of eating habits. Those already motivated can sometimes be helped by meeting as a group, when they can be given some nutrition education, helped to make their own decisions about dietary modifications, and given the opportunity to discuss mutual problems and support one another. Slimming clubs such as Weight Watchers can be helpful to slimmers.

When a satisfactory weight loss has been achieved dietary modifications can be cautiously relaxed. By means of trial and error it is possible to discover the degree of dietary relaxation consistent with the maintenance of a desirable weight.

Exceptionally strict diets

In selected cases which are slow to respond to dietary treatment the energy intake may be reduced to 2.5 or even 1.7 MJ daily (600 or 400 kcal). Such diets are normally prescribed only if the patient is in hospital where dietary discipline can be maintained and where the patient is under constant medical supervision. This treatment is seldom successful in the long term and is used as a last resort treatment, as is jaw wiring and jejunal by-pass surgery.

Proprietary foods and sweetening agents

Foods marketed as slimming agents, cannot substitute, in the long term, for re-education leading to a permanent change in eating habits. Soft drinks and confectionery intended for diabetics may be labelled as being free from sugar. They are not, however, necessarily suitable for those on reducing diets as they are often sweetened with a substitute sweetening agent, sorbitol, which has the same energy value as sugar. Other products such as low calorie soups, drinks and tinned fruits can add variety to diets which can become monotonous, and are convenient.

Drugs

Drugs which have the effect of reducing appetite may be of value in selected cases, for example diethylpropion (e.g. Tenuate Dospan, Merrell) and fenfluramine (Ponderax, Servier Laboratories Ltd). They are available only on prescription as they may give rise to uncomfortable or even serious side effects, including in some cases possible addiction to the drug itself. The amphetamines (e.g. Dexedrine) are no longer prescribed as aids to weight reduction as their abuse in the past has resulted in a high incidence of dependency. Preparations of methyl cellulose are sometimes added to the diet as this substance absorbs water and adds bulk to the gastric contents thus increasing the sense of satiety. This again should be taken only on the advice of a physician. It should not be forgotten that any benefit derived from drugs can only be temporary. For lasting effect a permanent change in eating habits is required.

DIET NO. 1 Suitable for the treatment of obesity

Energy value 4.2 MJ (1000 kcal) approximately

Suggested menu

Breakfast
Fruit or fruit juice.
Savoury, e.g. egg or sausage.
1 thin slice of wholemeal bread (30 g) with butter.
or
Helping of cereal e.g. 1 section Shredded Wheat with milk.
Coffee.

Mid-morning
Tea, coffee, Marmite or Bovril.

Mid-day meal
High protein serving:
e.g. average helping meat or fish (50–80 g) with large portions of vegetable such as carrot, turnip, or green leafy vegetable.
Some suggestions for alternative savoury dishes are given below.
1 small potato *or* 1 thick slice wholemeal bread.
Fruit, fresh, or stewed without the addition of sugar.
Coffee

Mid-afternoon
Tea

Evening meal
As at mid-day.

Allowances

Milk 250 ml full cream, or 500 ml skimmed milk daily.
Butter or margarine 15 g daily (100 g weekly).
 A little fat may be allowed in addition to this for the frying or grilling of fish, liver, or other non-starchy food.
Saccharine may be used for sweetening.

Savoury dishes — some suggested alternatives

The addition of cottage cheese to the salads will increase the food value without adding fat.

1. Salad with oil and vinegar dressing, using minimum oil. Good helping of lentil soup with one thick slice of bread toasted; no butter to be used on the bread if oil has been used in the salad dressing.

2. Salad as suggested above, or cooked vegetable such as cabbage. Spaghetti Bolognese.
 Omit the potato or bread.

3. Salad.
 1 thick slice bread toasted.
 A serving of baked beans in tomato sauce.

Foods to avoid

Sugar, glucose, syrup, honey, jam, marmalade and all preserves.
Sweets and chocolate. Diabetic confectionery, preserves and minerals.
Cakes, scones, puddings and pastry.
Soft drinks containing sugar. Ice cream.
Fried foods which have been coated with batter or crumbs.
Fried bread and fried potato.
Canned and dried fruit. Wine, beer and spirits.

Exchanges

The following foods are approximately equal in energy value:
170–250 kJ (40 to 60 kcal) and may be exchanged for one another.
1 slice wholemeal bread.
2 plain biscuits.
1 small potato.
3 tablespoons baked beans in tomato sauce.
3 tablespoons spaghetti rings in tomato sauce.
1 moderate serving of thickened soup such as bone and vegetable broth or cream of tomato.
1 serving fruit such as apple , banana, orange or pear.
2 tablespoons boiled rice.
1 carton natural yoghurt.

21

Diet following injury; pre-operative and post-operative diet; enteral and parenteral feeding

SUMMARY

1. It is important to maintain adequate nutritional intake following injury and to ensure that the patient remains in positive nitrogen balance.
2. Prior to surgery it is necessary for the patient to be as well nourished as possible. Following surgery it is important that food is re-introduced gradually.
3. Severely ill patients may receive nutritional support by nasogastric tube feeding or intravenous feeding if it is not possible to feed them orally.

Injuries, whether accidental or resulting from operative procedures, are followed by recovery which may be considered as taking place in two stages.

The period immediately following the injury is characterised by breakdown of body protein, giving rise to a state of negative nitrogen balance. Disturbance of fluid and electrolyte balance also occurs. The extent of these metabolic changes is proportional to the severity of the injury. For example, following the repair of a hernia the catabolic phase might be expected to last for only a few days, whereas in the case of a severely burned patient it can continue for ten days or more; even for some weeks if secondary infection occurs.

If this is a short period, there is nothing to be gained by giving a high protein diet as the patient usually has little or no desire for food. Treatment is therefore directed to maintaining fluid and electrolyte balance, by means of intravenous infusions if necessary, the nature of the diet being determined by the patient's appetite.

Following severe injuries such as major operations or extensive burns more active methods are required, and it is possible to mitigate the state of negative nitrogen balance if sufficient protein can be given, along with an adequate energy intake. In some cases a dietary supplement given by nasogastric tube is necessary. If this is impossible the patient may need to be fed parenterally.

During the second stage of convalescence protein replacement or anabolism takes place and the metabolic processes gradually return to normal. This period is characterised by weight increase and a renewed interest in food on the part of the patient. Care should be taken to provide a balanced diet. It is pointless to concentrate on protein alone, as an adequate energy intake from carbohydrate and fat is necessary if protein is to be available for tissue synthesis. High energy, high protein supplements should be given if necessary and an adequacy of ascorbic acid should be assured (30 mg/day). Food likes and dislikes should be carefully considered and meals should be attractively served. Unpleasant or painful procedures must on no account take place immediately before or following a meal and the patient should be comfortable and relaxed before being presented with food. The nurse must be prepared to offer much encouragement. It is important to assign an enthusiastic nurse to give individual attention to the very ill patient. In the post-operative period a weight increase of 1 to 1½ kg per week is an indication that the diet is adequate.

PRE-OPERATIVE DIET

Undernutrition

A healthy person, in a satisfactory state of nutrition, is in a favourable position to withstand the stress of an operation.

Undernourishment, however, is a feature of many conditions which require operative treatment, especially disorders of the alimentary tract. For example obstruction of the upper alimentary tract, such as might result from a malignant growth, may make an adequate food intake impossible. Gastric ulceration and its associated pain and discomfort may result in so many foods being avoided by the patient that the diet is inadequate. Inflammation and ulceration of the colon may result in the presence in the stools of mucus and blood, representing a loss to the body of protein and iron. In the case of a patient requiring plastic surgery for extensive burns there may be protein depletion due to loss of protein in the exudate from the surface of the burn.

A preliminary period of special feeding is of assistance in enabling the patient to make a satisfactory recovery. If this is done effectively, by intragastric tube or intravenous infusion if necessary, the operation can proceed with the minimum of delay.

Obesity

We have already seen that obese people are not good subjects for surgery as they present the surgeon with difficulties in diagnosis and of technique at the time of operation, and are prone to develop complications in the post-operative period. For these reasons a pre-operative period of weight reduction is frequently prescribed for patients awaiting elective surgery who are overweight. Details of a reducing regimen are given in Chapter 20.

The day of the operation

On the day of the operation no food is given unless the operation is a minor one and scheduled for late in the day, in which case the patient is allowed a light breakfast.

POST-OPERATIVE DIET

In many instances post-operative feeding presents no problems. The patient's appetite gradually returns and it only remains to ensure that a balanced diet is provided. Post-operatively the aim should be to provide, as soon as the patient can take it, a varied diet, adequate in protein content, and of sufficient energy value to spare the protein and permit a satisfactory weight gain in those patients who are under-nourished or who have lost much weight.

Following operations on the gastrointestinal tract, allowance must be made for a gradual resumption of intestinal motility, and the patient's basic needs are supplied intravenously, or sometimes directly into the jejunum, until it is possible to give an adequate food intake orally. At first water only is allowed by mouth in small amounts as prescribed by the surgeon, perhaps 30 ml hourly while the patient is awake. Amounts are gradually increased if tolerated. When the patient is taking free fluids a light diet of easily digested and non-bulky solids may be introduced. Gradually a normal diet is resumed. The length of time taken to return to a normal diet depends on the type of surgery, ie, gastrointestinal tract operations will take between 24 and 48 hours for bowel sounds to recur indicating the return of normal intestinal motility. Very little is absorbed from the bowel until its normal motility recommences. Any fluids taken will tend to pool, resulting in distension and nausea. This is why many patients will have a nasogastric tube which needs to be aspirated regularly until normal bowel activity returns. Once bowel sounds are heard and the volume of the nasogastric aspirates diminishes, then proper oral feeding can start in stages as indicated. Until then an adequate intake of fluid (2–3 litres per day) and electrolytes is given intravenously.

If the patient has had simple or minor surgery not involving the gastrointestinal tract they may eat as soon as they wish, but the effect the general anaesthetic may have had must be taken into account. Their appetite will be small initially. The general anaesthetic and possibly post-operative pain often tire the patient and may cause some nausea. A moderate light diet is best in the immediate post-operative period, however hungry the patient may feel.

ENTERAL AND PARENTERAL NUTRITION

Between 5 and 15 per cent of all patients admitted to hospital require some kind of nutritional support. This is indicated in all patients who should not, will not, or cannot eat because of their illness.

The types of patients who may require nutritional support are:

1. Pre-operative patients who, due to their disease, may be malnourished—these include those requiring gastrointestinal tract surgery, especially on the oesophagus and stomach.
2. Post-operative patients who develop complications and therefore may not be able to eat for some time following their surgery—possibly those with ileus.
3. Patients with disease of the gastrointestinal tract, such as inflammatory bowel disease or fistulae, who require bowel rest.
4. Patients with major trauma, burns or sepsis who need to be nursed in an intensive care unit.
5. Patients with neurological problems such as strokes or those who have had neurosurgery and whose conscious level is impaired.
6. Cancer patients who feel unable to eat sufficient and whose appetite may be reduced further during treatment with radiotherapy or cytotoxic drugs.

Patients can be fed in one of two ways.

Enteral nutrition is simpler, has fewer potential complications and is also the cheaper method. It involves feeding nutrients directly into the digestive tract through a nasogastric tube, a feeding jejunostomy or a gastrostomy. This is the normal way in which food enters the body. As long as there is no serious gastrointestinal disease, then this is the sensible natural route. *If the gut works use it!*

Parenteral nutrition can be used if enteral nutrition is impossible due to the condition of the patient or his disease. This involves infusing nutrients in a sterile purified state into a central vein. As it carries more potential complications, it should only be used when alternative methods are unsuitable.

ENTERAL NUTRITION

Systems and methods

In the past, tube feeds were usually administered by the bolus method, that is, a fixed amount of nutrient given at intervals throughout the day stopping overnight. However, a better method is to give the same amount steadily over a 24 hour period via a continuous gravity drip system. This delivers the feed at a slower rate and lessens the risk of problems such as nausea and diarrhoea. It has also become unnecessary to use starter regimes, that is, the building up in stages from $\frac{1}{4}$ to $\frac{1}{2}$ to full strength feed. A continuous flow system allows a fine bore 1 mm internal diameter PVC tube to be used which is simpler to manage and much more pleasant for the patient.

The tube is passed through the nose and into the stomach. Its position is checked by auscultating over the stomach as a bolus of air is injected and listening for bubbling through the gastric juice. Alternatively, an abdominal X-ray can be taken to check the position. This is illustrated in Figure 21.1.

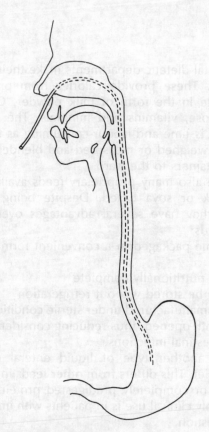

Figure 21.1 Positioning of fine bore tube.

It is not possible to aspirate through these tubes to check the gastric pH. These tubes are preferable to traditional Ryles tubes which, being considerably wider and made of a harder plastic, can cause nasopharyngeal and oesophageal ulceration.

The tube is connected to a standard delivery system which consists of a reservoir to hold the feed of 1–2 litre capacity sufficient for 12–24 hours. This is connected via a giving set to the fine bore tube and the rate adjusted to deliver 1–2 ml per minute over the 24 hour period. Although the flow rate needs to be checked regularly, this method minimises nursing time spent in administering feeds. Numerous feeding tubes and delivery systems are available. Where possible one system should be used throughout the hospital. All connections in enteral giving systems are incompatible with intravenous systems.

Feeds

Many hospital dietetic departments make their own standard tube feeds. These provide calories from protein, fat and carbohydrate in the form of milk powder, Complan, Prosporol, glucose, vitamins and minerals. The preparation of these feeds is time and labour-consuming as the ingredients have to be weighed or measured and blended before being sent in containers to the ward.

There are also many proprietary feeds available which are usually milk or soya based. Despite being comparatively expensive they have several advantages over the standard hospital feeds:
1. They come packaged in a convenient form for immediate use
2. They are nutritionally complete
3. They can be stored without refrigeration
4. They are manufactured under sterile conditions and remain sterile until opened, thus reducing considerably the risk of gastrointestinal infections.

There is another type of liquid enteral diet called an elemental diet. This differs from other feeds in that it consists of partially or completely predigested protein and carbohydrate. Its only clinical use is in patients with impaired absorption or digestion.

Table 21.1 Some proprietary enteric feeds

Product	Manufacturer	Palatable	Nitrogen source	Quantity	Energy (kcals)	Protein (g)	Fat (g)	Na (mmol)	K (mmol)	Ca (mmol)	Mg (mmol)	P (mmol)
Complan	Farley-Health Products Ltd	yes	whole protein	100 g	444	20	16	15.2	21.8	18.3	2.9	18.7
Clinifeed 400	Roussel Labs Ltd	yes	whole protein	375 ml (1 can)	400	15	13.4	10.5	12.4	5.0	2.0	7.4
Ensure	Abbott Labs Ltd	yes	whole protein	235 ml (1 can)	241	8.7	8.7	7.6	7.7	3.1	2.0	1.6
Isocal	Mead Johnson Labs	no	whole protein	355 ml (1 can)	375	12.1	15.7	8.1	12	5.6	3.1	6.1
Triosorbon	F Merck Ltd	yes	whole protein	85 g (1 pkt)	400	16.2	16.2	17	17	5.1	3	7.7
Flexical	Mead Johnson Labs	yes	oligopeptides + free amino acids	100 g (1 can)	441	9.9	15	6.7	14.1	6.6	3.7	7.1
Vivonex Standard	Eaton Labs	no	free amino acids	80 g (1 pkt)	300	6.3	4	11.2	9	3.3	2.4	1.4
Vivonex HN	Eaton Labs	no	free amino acids	80 g (1 pkt)	300	12.5	0.3	10.1	5.4	2.0	1.4	0.8

All these products can be given as a tube feed or as an oral supplement. The composition of the elemental diets makes them generally unpalatable although flavourings are available to improve the taste. Table 21.1 gives examples of the constituents of some of these feeds.

High protein and high energy supplements

Patients who are unable to maintain sufficient oral intake of food may require supplements to their diet in the form of high protein liquids. This group would include patients with long-term infection and fever who do not feel well enough to eat a normal diet.

Infection will increase the basal metabolic rate, resulting in increased energy expenditure. Protein requirement is also increased as without sufficient intake, the body stores of glycogen, fat and tissue protein will be utilised, resulting in weight loss and tissue wastage.

Fluid intake has to be sufficient especially if the patient is sweating profusely which may result in reduced urinary output.

1. If the patient is taking liquid supplements in addition to normal hospital food it should be ensured that small portions of easily digested food are given at frequent intervals.

2. The diet should be high in energy giving 2000–2500 calories daily either by food and supplements, or supplements alone.

3. Protein intake should be high to counteract breakdown of body tissue. Milk and eggs provide protein in a palatable and easily digested form. They can be given in a variety of ways, e.g., soups, jellies, custards, junket and egg flips.

4. A liberal intake of carbohydrate in the form of glucose may be given. As it is easily tolerated and soluble it can be added to milk drinks, fruit juice and jellies.

5. Fat in the form of cream can be added to junkets, jellies, soups and cereals as it makes a valuable contribution to the energy requirement.

6. Fluid intake should be at least $2\frac{1}{2}$ litres per day. This is roughly equivalent to 160 ml hourly for 16 hours of the 24 whilst the patient is awake.

The responsibility for ensuring that requirements are met

falls upon the nurse, as these patients require constant encouragement.

Types of high energy and high protein supplements

Caloreen (Roussel Laboratory Ltd) and *Maxijul* (Scientific Hospital Supplies Ltd) are examples of a manufactured carbohydrate yielding glucose on digestion and supplying 4 calories per g. They are virtually tasteless and due to their molecular structure are less likely to cause diarrhoea than either cane sugar or glucose when given in concentrated solution. They have a low electrolyte content and are suitable for situations when sodium and potassium intakes are restricted as in renal failure.

Prosparol (Duncan Flockhart & Co Ltd) is a palatable oil and water emulsion of the same energy value as double cream. It may be given without modification or added to soups, milk or fruit juices.

Dried milk powders consist of the solid constituents of the milk from which practically all of the water has been removed. Full cream and skimmed milk powders are available. They may be mixed with water to the required concentration or added to fresh milk. They may also be added to milk puddings, soups, etc. Full cream milk powder supplies 26 g protein and 490 calories per 100 g.

Carnation build-up (Carnation Foods Co Ltd) contains as its major ingredients skimmed milk solids, sucrose, vitamins and minerals. It is in powder form and is available in a variety of flavours and is added to milk to make a flavoured drink. It contains 22.4 per cent protein and the fat content is minimal, making it suitable for use with skimmed milk in low fat diets.

Complan (Farley Health Products) supplies approximately 20 g protein and 444 calories per 100 g. It contains the protein, fat, carbohydrate, vitamins and minerals of a balanced diet. It may be mixed with water or milk to make a palatable and nourishing drink.

Casilan (Farley Health Products) contains approximately 90 per cent protein derived from milk. It is of particular value when a high protein intake is required. Another advantage, especially for patients with renal disease, is that it contains only 7 mg sodium per 100 g.

Hycal (Beecham Products) is a high carbohydrate, low elec-trolyte, low fluid drink. It supplies 415 calories per bottle and again is suitable for patients suffering from renal disease.

PARENTERAL NUTRITION

Parenteral feeding should only be implemented if it is not possible to feed the patient by the enteral route. Once it has been decided to feed a patient parenterally a central venous line is inserted under aseptic conditions, preferably in the operating theatre.

Silicone catheters are best because they cause fewer long-term problems. The subclavian vein is cannulated following the normal procedure for insertion of a central venous line. The only difference is that the line is then tunnelled under the skin and out onto the chest wall. Using this method the exit point is separated from the venous entry site lessening the risk of infection, as shown in Figure 21.2.

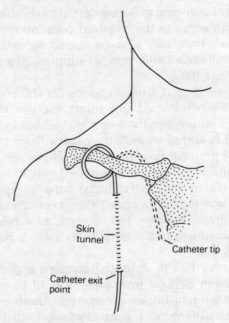

Skin tunnel

Catheter tip

Catheter exit point

Figure 21.2 Positioning of tunnelled central feeding line.

The area is easy to keep clean and the flat surface of the chest wall is more suitable for dressing. It is also more comfortable for the patient and does not restrict his mobility. Maintenance of sterility is absolutely essential in the nursing and general care of parenteral feeding lines. The site should be cleaned and redressed every 2–5 days as necessary and all intravenous tubing changed daily.

The line should only be used for the infusion of nutritional products. Blood must not be withdrawn from the line nor blood transfusions given through it. Under no circumstances should central venous pressure measurements be taken, as this increases the risk of infection.

Administration of parenteral solutions

Prescribed solutions can be given through a two or three line system running several bottles of amino acid, electrolyte, dextrose and lipid solutions simultaneously, but this is difficult to manage and monitor. A much better method is to use a 3 litre bag with all the solutions ready mixed in it. These bags are made up daily under sterile conditions using a laminar flow hood in the hospital pharmacy. The contents of the bag are then infused via a single giving set over a 24 hour period. The system is further simplified by using a volumetric pump to infuse a measured amount steadily each hour. This is illustrated in Figure 21.3.

Solutions

Nitrogen source

Protein is given in the form of pure amino acid solutions. It has already been pointed out in Chapter 4 that certain amino acids are essential components of the diet as they cannot be synthesised in the body. In total parenteral nutrition all essential amino acids must be provided and must be present at the same time.

A sufficient amount of energy in the form of carbohydrate must be available simultaneously otherwise the protein will be used as an energy source instead of being incorporated into body proteins.

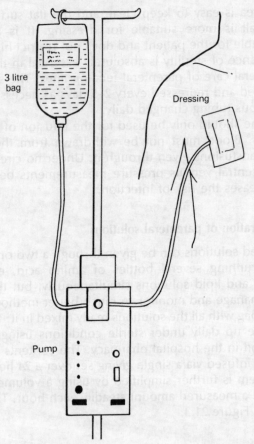

3 litre bag

Dressing

Pump

Figure 21.3 3 litre bag and pump on patient receiving parenteral nutrition.

Energy sources

Hypertonic glucose is a suitable source of carbohydrate. As solutions of glucose which are more concentrated than the normal 5 per cent isotonic solution are irritant to peripheral veins, it is essential that hypertonic glucose is infused through a central vein.

In stress situations, notably surgical operations, severe burns and hypothermia, endogenous insulin secretion may be insufficient. If the patient becomes hyperglycaemic insulin is infused along with the carbohydrate.

Table 21.2 Some solutions containing nitrogen source for parenteral nutrition (Constituents per litre)

Solution	Manufacturer	kcal	N(g)	Na	K	Mg	Ca	P
Aminoplex 14	Geistlich	340	13.4	35	30	—	—	—
Synthamin 9	Travenol	250	9.3	73	60	5	—	30
Synthamin 14	Travenol	375	14.3	73	60	5	—	30
Synthamin 17	Travenol	450	16.9	73	60	5	—	30
Vamin N	Kabivitrum	250	9.4	50	20	1.5	2.5	—
Vamin glucose	Kabivitrum	650	9.4	50	20	1.5	2.5	—

Fat solutions have a high energy content relative to volume; therefore, they are invaluable in total parenteral nutrition. A common 10 per cent solution contains 1000 kcal per litre.

Electrolytes, trace elements and vitamins

In total parenteral nutrition, provision of electrolytes, trace elements and vitamins must be comprehensive and complete. Some solutions used may already contain electrolytes but additions can be made as necessary. Sodium and potassium are especially important where there are large gastrointestinal losses, for example, as a result of vomiting, diarrhoea or substantial gastric aspiration. Visible sweating is another route for large losses of sodium.

Table 21.3 Some solutions containing the calorie source for parenteral nutrition (constituents per litre)

Solution	Manufacturer	kcal	N(g)	Na	K	Mg	Ca	P
Polyfusor (20% dextrose)	Boots	800	—	—	—	—	—	—
Polyfusor (50% dextrose)	Boots	2000	—	—	—	—	—	—
Electrolyte Solution A (with 20% dextrose)	Travenol	800	—	—	—	28	26	—
Electrolyte Solution B (with 20% dextrose)	Travenol	800	—	—	60	—	—	60
Intralipid 10%	Kabivitrum	1000	—	—	—	—	—	15
Intralipid 20%	Kabivitrum	2000	—	—	—	—	—	15

The trace elements cobalt, copper, fluoride, iodine, iron, magnesium and zinc are all important for human metabolism and can be added to intravenous nutrients satisfactorily. Addamel contains calcium and chloride, whilst at the same time giving the daily requirements of trace elements.

Patients receiving intravenous feeding require increased vitamin supplements as they are excreted rapidly from the body. Solivito contains the water soluble vitamin B group and vitamin C.

Vitlipid is a fat emulsion to be added to Intralipid containing the fat soluble vitamins A, D and K.

Some solutions used in parenteral feeding and their constituents are shown in Tables 21.2 and 21.3.

Nitrogen balance

With the administration of all types of feeds the aim is for the patients to ingest more nitrogen than they excrete, that is, to maintain a positive nitrogen balance (see Ch. 4). This is estimated by daily 24 h urine collections, measuring urea and creatinine levels. Adjustments to nitrogen intake are made as necessary and positive nitrogen balance is maintained.

Protein energy requirements

Estimated daily needs:

	Protein (g)	Energy (kcal)
Medical patient	45–75	1500–2000
Surgical patient	75–125	3000
Hypercatabolic patient	125–200	3500

Patient monitoring

Blood urea and electrolytes are measured to indicate renal function and allow sodium and potassium supplements to be given if necessary. Liver enzymes are measured to monitor any liver damage, and serum albumin to establish the extent of hepatic protein synthesis.

Parenterally fed patients, because of the high dextrose content of the feed have to have regular blood and urine sugar checks to detect hyperglycaemia. If necessary insulin may be added to the 3 litre bag to control blood sugar levels.

A strict fluid balance chart must be kept for all patients. In order to monitor their recovery patients must be weighed twice weekly.

Nutrition team

Ideally, the feeding of patients in hospital, either enterally or parenterally, should be supervised by a nutrition team consisting of doctors, nurses, dietitians, pharmacists and biochemists. Using this multi-disciplinary approach, the condition of patients can be monitored and discussed with other team members who can use their individual expertise to optimise nutritional support for the patient.

Medical and nursing staff are involved at a practical level in the patient's daily care. They will determine the individual nutritional requirements for that day and discuss them with the dietitians and pharmacists who prepare the enteral and parenteral feeds. The biochemist monitors the patient's metabolic state by analysing blood, urine and other samples which are taken regularly. He can often give an early warning of metabolic imbalances which can then be corrected.

The main aim of the nutrition team is to work together to simplify clinical nutrition for the ward staff, and they are available for the practical care and advice on this aspect of the patient's treatment. Ideally, they should provide a service throughout the hospital. The procedures can then be standardised throughout all units and wards. This avoids confusion for the other staff involved in caring for those patients receiving nutritional support.

Home feeding

It is possible for patients with long-term feeding problems to receive nutritional support at home. Once they are familiar with the equipment and procedures for enteral or parenteral feeding and providing they receive adequate back-up services from both the hospital nutrition team and community services, they usually encounter few problems. The types of patient who receive nutritional support at home are usually cases of inflammatory bowel disease or ischaemic bowel disease who have had total bowel resection and are therefore unable to eat normally. As these patients have chronic conditions, they require long-term nutrition. The most satisfactory method is to train them to manage their own parenteral feeding at home.

CASE HISTORY—ENTERAL FEEDING 1

Day 0   19-year-old male
Admitted with head injury and multiple fractures
Required ventilation following surgery therefore
Nursed in Intensive Care Unit
No internal injuries

Day 3   Bowel sounds present
Fine bore tube passed
Nitrogen requirement high
Commenced on:
2 litres of feed
  3000 calories
  114 g protein   Given over 24 hrs
  117 g fat
  375 g carbohydrate
  + all necessary trace elements, minerals and vitamins

Day 10   Ventilation no longer required
Conscious level improving
Nitrogen requirement less
Feed reduced to:
2 litres
  2000 calories
  60 g protein   Given over 24 hours
  85 g fat
  250 g carbohydrate

Day 12   Commenced oral liquid supplements
Continues on 2 litre, 2000 calorie feed

Day 14   Transferred to general ward
Oral intake improved
Taking normal ward diet
Fine bore tube removed.

CASE HISTORY—ENTERAL FEEDING 2

Day 0   73-year-old female
Admitted following a cerebrovascular accident
Semiconscious without a gag reflex
Initial resuscitation with intravenous fluids

Day 2   Fine bore feeding tube passed
Commenced on enteral feeding:
2 litres
  2000 calories
  60 g protein   Given over 24 hours
  85 g fat
  250 g carbohydrate
  + All necessary vitamins, minerals and trace elements

Day 6   Remains stable
Still no gag reflex
Continues on 2 litre, 2000 calorie feed

Day 13   More alert
Swallowing improved—taking sips of fluids
Maintained on 2 litre, 2000 calorie feed

Day 18   Continues to improve
Taking 500–800 ml oral liquid supplements daily
Enteral feed reduced to:
1 litre
  1000 calories
  30 g protein   Given over 12 hours at night
  42 g fat
  125 g carbohydrate

Day 23   Now taking soft hospital diet + liquid supplements
Fine bore tube removed

CASE HISTORY: PARENTERAL FEEDING 1

Day 0   50-year-old male
Ten days post-oesophagogastrectomy
Has developed leak in anastomosis
Nil by mouth
Needs parenteral nutrition
Central venous line inserted in theatre

Day 1   Commenced on 3 litres total parenteral nutrition (TPN)
consisting of:

Amino acid solution containing 14 g nitrogen	1000 ml
50% dextrose	500 ml
Electrolyte solution (in 20% dextrose)	1000 ml
20% lipid solution	500 ml

+ trace elements, minerals and vitamins
  1000 i.u. heparin to prevent clotting in the line
  24 units Actrapid insulin to keep blood sugar under control
Sodium and potassium levels were adjusted according to serum
electrolyte results.
This regime gave a total of 2800 calories.

Day 2–9   Continues on same regime
Adjustments for serum electrolytes and blood glucose made as
required

Day 10   Barium swallow performed
Anastomosis now healed
Oral fluids commenced
TPN to continue until sufficient food orally

QUESTIONS

1. Explain nitrogen balance and how is is achieved.
2. Detail the stages in which oral feeding is recommenced following surgery.
3. Name five types of patient who may require nutritional support.
4. What is the difference between enteral and parenteral nutrition?
5. When do patients require high protein and high energy supplements?

22

Diet in disorders of the cardiovascular system

SUMMARY

Diet is important in the prevention and treatment of cardiovascular disease. The role of diet in the prevention of cardiovascular disease is discussed in Chapter 9.

Patients with cardiovascular disease have raised blood lipids and are often obese. In order that they lose weight, the energy content of the diet of obese patients is restricted. The raised blood lipid levels are corrected by a reduction in the total amount and modification of the type of fat eaten.

Modifications of the diet in disorders of the heart and circulatory system are based on three principles:

1. The energy value of the diet is reduced if the patient is overweight.

2. When oedema is present it is usual to use diuretics to reduce the extracellular fluid volume. The volume of extracellular fluid is determined by its sodium content. Diuretics prevent the reabsorption of sodium by the renal tubules. It is sometimes necessary to restrict dietary sodium intake as a supplementary measure.

3. Both the total amount of fat in the diet and the proportion provided by saturated fats are reduced when the serum lipids are raised. If the cholesterol-containing lipid fraction is raised the dietary intake of cholesterol is restricted.

ATHEROSCLEROSIS

Atherosclerosis is the underlying cause of cardiovascular disease. Fatty deposits develop in the lining of the inner wall of the artery. These grow and become covered with fibrous connective tissue. This narrows the inner channel of the blood vessel and so slows the flow of blood through it. It also reduces the elasticity of the blood vessel. When the coronary arteries become atherosclerotic, blood flow to the heart is reduced and coronary heart disease (ischaemic heart disease) develops. Atherosclerosis can also damage the main arteries of the legs and affect the brain, causing a stroke.

A mild degree of atherosclerosis is common among adults in Western countries. The incidence of more severe atherosclerosis causing coronary heart disease and stroke is high, so high that the chance of a man aged 40 having a heart attack before is is 65 are 1 in 5.

WEIGHT REDUCTION

It is important to avoid obesity in cardiovascular disorders. Excessive weight gain puts an added burden on the heart, and deposits of a fat in the heart muscle itself may impair its efficiency. Large amounts of fat around the abdominal organs may interfere with respiration by impeding the movements of the diaphragm. This aggravates the breathlessness of heart disease. Some physicians prefer that the patient should be slightly underweight. Modification of the diet for weight reduction is discussed in detail in Chapter 20.

SODIUM RESTRICTION

Dietary sources of sodium

1. Sodium is a natural constituent of all foodstuffs. On the

whole meat, fish, milk and eggs contain more sodium than do fruits, cereals and vegetables.

2. Sodium is a constituent of common salt (sodium chloride) used in cooking and at the table as a condiment. It is also a component of monosodium glutamate, used for flavouring savoury dishes, and items such as stock cubes.

3. The sodium content of food is increased by various methods of preservation involving the addition of salt, for example the preparation of ham, tongue, and other salt meats, the preservation of fish, and the preparation of cheese, chutneys, pickles, bottled sauces and canned and salted vegetables.

4. Baking soda (sodium bicarbonate), which is extensively used as a raising agent and is a constituent of baking powders, contributes sodium to the diet.

Diets restricted in sodium

In most cases a moderate degree of restriction as outlined by Diet No. 2 below is sufficient. The diet may also be used to treat primary hypertension. In some people hypertension is associated with a high dietary salt intake.

Most diuretic drugs promote excretion of potassium, as well as that of sodium. To prevent potassium depletion during diuretic therapy supplements of this mineral may be required.

DIET NO. 2 No-added-salt diet.

The following modifications of a normal diet are required:
1. A minimum of salt should be used in cooking.
2. Salt should not be added to food at the table.
3. Milk intake should be restricted to 500 ml daily.
4. The following foods should be avoided:
   Obviously salty foods such as bacon, ham, tongue, sausages, canned meat and fish, smoked fish, cheese, meat and fish pastes. Canned vegetables, canned tomato juice, pickles, chutneys, sauces and ketchups. Canned and packet soups.
   Meat and yeast extracts. Stock cubes. Foods listed as containing salt, or monosodium glutamate.

Table 22.1 The sodium content of portions of salty foods

Food	mg sodium
60 g (2 oz) cheddar cheese	370
30 g (1 slice) tinned ham	375
1 packet salted potato crisps	165
3 g (thin spreading) marmite	135

FAT RESTRICTION

In atherosclerosis a high level of blood cholesterol may be observed.

Studies comparing populations in different parts of the world have shown that high blood cholesterol levels are one of a number of factors which are associated with an increased incidence of coronary heart disease. The condition is also associated with the consumption of a high proportion of saturated fats, such as are found in dairy produce, eggs and meat, as compared with unsaturated fats, which are present in oils.

It is possible to bring about a reduction of blood cholesterol level by reducing the intake of fats. This is accomplished by eating less of the fatty foods—cheese, butter, cream, margarine, pastry, cakes, fatty meat—and by not frying food. Fat-containing foods have a high energy value. A reduction in fat intake results in a decreased energy intake and weight loss. If obesity is not present extra food in the form of unrefined carbohydrate should be included in the diet. For example extra bread without butter.

In some situations it is also necessary to reduce the dietary intake of cholesterol. Cholesterol is found in animal fats. Egg yolks are the major source of cholesterol in the United Kingdom diet—one egg yolk contains 250 mg cholesterol. Other foods which are rich sources of cholesterol are milk, cheese, cream, butter, offal and shell fish. Cholesterol is also synthesised in the body. It is incorporated into hormones and bile salts and is found in the fatty covering of nerves and in the brain. Dietary cholesterol intake is controlled by:
1. limiting egg yolks to two a week

2. substituting skimmed milk for whole milk,
3. substituting vegetable fats for animal fats
4. avoiding cholesterol-rich foods.

There is some evidence to suggest that increasing the proportion of fat provided as polyunsaturated fatty acids is beneficial. Diet No. 3 is high in polyunsaturated fats and low in cholesterol.

DIET NO. 3 High in unsaturated fatty acids and low in cholesterol

1. Skimmed milk should be substituted for full cream milk.
2. Ordinary butter, margarine and cooking fats should be avoided. Corn oil may be used for cooking and for dressing salads. For baking and at the table special margarines high in unsaturated fatty acids are available. Examples are Flora (Van den Berghs) and Golden Corn (Kraft Foods Ltd.)
3. (a) As far as possible lean cuts of meat should be selected. Visible fat should be removed.
   (b) Fish may be substituted for lean meat as desired. White fish have a low fat content, while the oil which is present in the tissues of dark-fleshed or fatty fish is largely unsaturated.
   (c) As egg yolk has particularly high contents of cholesterol and saturated fat it is important not to exceed the allowance of two. Egg white is unrestricted.
   (d) Cheese should be avoided, with the exception of cottage cheese, which may be taken in unrestricted amounts.

Foods to avoid

Some items which should be avoided are given above; in addition, the following:
Offal, such as liver and kidney.
Pastry and cakes containing eggs, and fats and other than those permitted.
Confectionery containing fat, for example chocolate and toffee. Ice cream.

PREVENTION

The relationships between diet and cardiovascular disease are currently the subject of much research. Many authorities feel that the evidence is sufficient to justify dietary modifications to prevent cardiovascular disease as well as to help those suffering from it. The dietary recommendations to prevent cardiovascular disease are:

1. maintain ideal body weight
2. reduce total fat intake
3. reduce salt intake.

The importance of other nutrients including fibre, animal protein and sugar are still under debate.

QUESTIONS

1. What is atherosclerosis?
2. How can the diet be modified to lower raised serum lipids?
3. Suggest a day's meals which are both low in cholesterol and fat and are palatable.

23

Diet in disorders of the gastrointestinal tract

SUMMARY

1. When the digestive and absorptive functions of the gastrointestinal tract are impaired by disease, dietary treatment is often necessary to provide nutrients in forms which can be digested and absorbed and so avoid malabsorption.

2. Essential nutrients which cannot be absorbed adequately can be replaced with supplements.

3. The most commonly used diet for gastrointestinal disorders is the high fibre diet. Increasing the fibre content of the diet is the most successful treatment for chronic constipation.

4. Many disorders of the gastrointestinal tract require no specific dietary treatment. Patients with these disorders benefit from the advice to eat a varied diet and avoid foods which upset them.

INTRODUCTION

Better understanding of the physiology of the gastrointestinal tract, new and improved treatments for alimentary disorders and a critical appraisal of the effectiveness of the previously prescribed diets have led to changes in the dietetic treatment of disorders of the gastrointestinal tract. Diets used in the past, such as the Salisbury diet, based on lean meat and hot water, used for the treatment of dyspepsia, and the Sippy diet for ulcers consisting of hourly feeds of milk and cream, are now obsolete.

Despite this progress, most patients expect to be given dietary advice. To them, it seems obvious that the food they eat will affect their condition. The conditions which require specific dietary modifications are outlined in this chapter. The best advice for patients where no special advice is necessary is:

Eat a simple varied diet

Avoid the foods that upset you.

PEPTIC ULCER AND DYSPEPSIA

Dyspepsia, that is, meal-related indigestion-like pain, is a common symptom. In many instances, it is unrelated to detectable diseases of the gastrointestinal tract. However, in a proportion of patients with dyspepsia, ulceration of inflammation of the lining of the gut will be found.

Ulceration of the upper part of the alimentary tract which comes into contact with acid gastric juice is known as peptic ulceration. The factors responsible for the development of peptic ulcers are not fully understood. It is believed that they are caused by digestion of the mucosa by the gastric acid and pepsin, often in association with impairment of this membrane's protective mechanisms. Excessive secretion of hydrochloric acid may be a contributing factor. Peptic ulceration is sometimes associated with emotional stress.

Treatment with antacids will relieve symptoms and will help ulcers to heal. Newer specific anti-ulcer drugs such as histamine H_2-receptor antagonists reduce acid production and greatly improve the healing rate of the ulcer.

Principles of dietary treatment

These are summarised in the Table below. The dietary modifications should incorporate the minimum of restrictions and interfere as little as possible with the eating habits of the patients.

---

1. Take a snack at bedtime and between meals
2. Avoid foods that upset you, highly spiced food and alcohol

---

1. Food in the stomach buffers the acid gastric juice and stimulates the production of bicarbonate rich pancreatic secretion which neutralises acid in the duodenum. Patients usually feel more comfortable if they eat small, frequent meals.

2. Some foods, particularly alcohol and highly spiced foods, are gastric irritants and are best avoided.

Acute oesophagitis, gastritis and duodenitis

These may occur without mucosal ulceration though they produce similar symptoms. They are treated according to the same principles as peptic ulcer. Common causes of gastritis are the ingestion of gastric irritants such as alcohol and the excessive use of anti-inflammatory and analgesic drugs.

The dumping syndrome following gastric surgery

A small proportions of patients who have a surgical procedure designed to increase the rate of drainage of the stomach, suffer from symptoms which develop shortly after taking food. These may include faintness, muscular weakness, epigastric discomfort, giddiness and sweating. In the majority of cases, symptoms gradually disappear or lessen in severity, but in a few they persist. In some instances, symptoms are alleviated if the patient lies down for half an hour after taking food.

There are two types of dumping syndrome, early and late, which are caused by different mechanisms. The rapid emptying of the hypertonic stomach contents into the small bowel is, however, the common factor in both types.

Early dumping occurs within 30 minutes of eating a meal. The rapid passage of the hypertonic meal draws large amounts of fluid into the intestine. This causes a decrease in the circulating plasma volume, and it is this that produces the early symptoms of faintness, weakness, distension and discomfort.

Dietary advice for early dumping:
1. Eat small frequent dry meals
2. Take drinks *between*, not *with* meals
3. Avoid foods which worsen symptoms.

Late dumping occurs 1½–2 hours after a meal. A rapid rise in blood glucose follows the rapid gastric emptying. This stimulates an overproduction of insulin which causes a rapid drop in blood glucose and the symptoms of hypoglycaemia.

Dietary advice for late dumping:
1. Avoid sugar and sugar-containing foods
2. Eat carbohydrate as starch instead of sugar
3. Avoid foods which worsen symptoms.

Long-term complications of gastric surgery

Following gastric surgery, absorption of some essential nutrients, such as iron, folic acid, vitamin B_{12}, vitamins B, D and K and calcium, may occur. These present as late nutritional deficiencies and can be treated by providing dietary supplements.

Atrophic gastritis

Atrophic gastritis does not produce abdominal symptoms but causes a macrocytic anaemia due to vitamin B_{12} malabsorption. This is of nutritional importance because, along with the acid and pepsin-secreting cells, the cells which produce the intrinsic factor necessary for vitamin B_{12} absorption atrophy. So these patients are likely to develop a deficiency of this vitamin and require B_{12} injections to prevent this.

CONSTIPATION AND DIARRHOEA

In the United Kingdom each year, five million prescriptions for laxatives and purgatives are written and 40 000 gallons of liquid paraffin are drunk. Delay and difficulty in evacuation of faeces is known as constipation. This usually occurs because the stool is either too hard or its volume is small. In most cases constipation is not related to any organic disease but due to long established habits and a diet that is deficient in dietary fibre. When the diet lacks fibre the faeces are not bulky enough to be passed effectively by normal peristalsis. This results in an increase in the activity of the muscles of the colon, colonic spasm and chronic constipation. Diarrhoea is a less common symptom than constipation but can be equally troublesome. Diarrhoea means the passage, often frequent, of loose and bulky stools (usually more than 200 ml/day).

Constipation

Constipation is a rare condition in areas where there is a high intake of dietary fibre. The use of laxative and aperient drugs can be avoided in many cases of constipation by treatment with a high fibre diet. Different people require different amounts of fibre in their diet. An adequate amount of fibre is the amount required to allow the patient to pass a soft stool without effort.

Table 23.1 Fibre content of food portions

Food	Fibre content (g)
1 slice white bread	1
1 slice wholemeal bread	3.5
portion of corn flakes	1.5
portion of All Bran	10
or	
2 Weetabix	5
1 orange	2
portion of baked beans	5

DIET NO. 4

The fibre content of the diet can be increased by making the following simple dietary changes:

1. Eat a whole grain or bran enriched breakfast cereal, for example, Weetabix, Puffed Wheat, Shredded Wheat, or All Bran.
2. Eat wholemeal bread instead of white bread and eat more of it.
3. Eat more fruit and vegetables.
4. Avoid refined cereal products, for example, cakes, biscuits,

polished rice and pasta. Use whole grain products and brown rice instead.

The fibre content of some portions of foods are listed in Table 23.1.

The way in which the meals eaten in one day can be altered to increase their fibre content is shown in Table 23.2.

Table 23.2 Ways of increasing fibre content of a typical diet

Typical diet (low in fibre)	Fibre content (g)	Suggested diet (high in fibre)	Fibre content (g)
Grapefruit juice		Grapefruit	2
Cornflakes and milk	1.5	Shredded wheat and milk	6
2 slices white toast, butter and honey	2	2 slices wholemeal toast, butter and chunky marmalade	7
Cheese sandwiches (4 slices white bread)	4	Cheese sandwiches (4 slices wholemeal bread)	14
Fruit yoghurt		Tomato	1
		1 orange	2
Lamb chop		Lamb chop	
Boiled potato	1	Potato baked in jacket	2
Carrots	3	Carrots	3
		Peas	3
Fruit pie (made with white flour)	2	Fruit pie (made with wholemeal flour)	4
Custard		Custard	
Daily total	13.5	Daily total	44

If these dietary changes are not sufficient to relieve constipation, then extra fibre in the form of wheat bran must be taken. Again, there is individual variation about the amount required but most people need 6–10 teaspoons of bran a day. A tablespoonful of bran contains approximately 2 g of fibre. Bran is dry, fibrous and unpalatable so should not be taken on its own. It is best taken divided between the day's meals where it can be mixed into cereal, stewed fruits, yoghurt, soups and gravy and used in baking. A sudden increase in the amount of fibre taken in the diet may result in distension, discomfort and flatulence. To minimise these it is best to start at a low dose and increase fibre gradually to the level which the patient can take comfortably. At first, two teaspoons of bran should be incorporated into meals twice a day and the amount of bran gradually increased until the symptoms of constipation are relieved.

Diverticular disease and diverticulitis

A colonic diverticulum is formed when the colonic mucosa is pushed through the colonic muscle wall to form a blind sac. These are commonly found in people who have a low fibre diet resulting in small hard stools which require increased colonic muscular activity for their passage. The presence of asymptomatic diverticula, known as diverticular disease, increases with age. These diverticula are usually multiple.

Age group	% population with diverticular disease
31–50	9
51–70	36
71+	56

The mechanism of formation of a diverticulum is illustrated schematically in Figure 23.1.

The symptomatic form of diverticular disease is called acute diverticulitis and is due to acute inflammation of an obstructed diverticulum. After treatment of the acute inflammation, the traditional management was with a low fibre diet and liquid paraffin. Treatment is now completely different and based on increasing rather than decreasing the amount of fibre in the diet. Dietary recommendations are those for the treatment of constipation, as discussed above.

Diarrhoea

Acute diarrhoea has many causes, the commonest being dietary indiscretion and bacterial food poisoning. It is usually mild and does not require dietary treatment though generous fluids and a simple light diet probably speed recovery.

Chronic diarrhoea can be caused by:

1. Diseases of the gastrointestinal tract such as ulcerative

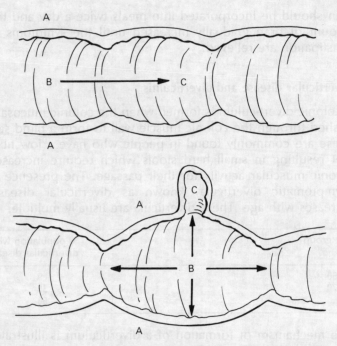

Figure 23.1 Normal colonic movement. (*Upper*) contraction of the colonic segment at A propels colonic contents B into C. (*Lower*) If the colonic contents are small and hard this cannot occur. Instead pressures build up in B, the result being the herniation of the colonic wall and the formation of a diverticulum at C.

colitis, Crohn's disease and sometimes carcinoma of the colon.
2. Malabsorption
3. Excessive alcohol consumption
4. The action of toxins as, for example, in uraemia.

The symptoms may be severe enough to require fluid and electrolyte replacement. Management involves treatment of the underlying disorder, and with dietary supplements for any nutritional deficienceis that have developed as a consequence of the diarrhoea. In some cases of intractable diarrhoea, a low residue diet may be used.

Foods to avoid on a low residue diet

Bread and biscuits made from brown or wholemeal flours

Breakfast cereals which contain the whole grain or are forti-
fied with bran.
Seeds and skins of fruit
Fruit which has a specific laxative effect–prunes, rhubarb
Pulses and fibrous vegetables.

THE IRRITABLE BOWEL SYNDROME

Symptoms coming from the bowel in the absence of detectable organic disease are described as the irritable bowel
syndrome. Between 25 and 30 per cent of referrals to gastroenterology clinics are eventually diagnosed as having irritable
bowel syndrome. It commonly presents with abdominal pain
and a variety of other symptoms which include constipation,
diarrhoea, alternating constipation and diarrhoea, flatulence,
heartburn, anorexia, nausea and occasionally vomiting.

Dietary treatment

There is no specific dietary treatment — some patients' symptoms are relieved by a high fibre diet, others by a low fibre
diet. Emphasis should be placed on eating a varied diet
avoiding the foods which aggravate the individual's condition.

MALABSORPTION SYNDROMES

Malabsorption of nutrients results from a wide range of
diseases and disorders of the gastrointestinal tract. Generally,
if the disorder reduces enzyme secretion or damages the sites
of nutrient absorption,malabsorption is the result. The symptoms of malabsorption include diarrhoea, steatorrhoea,
abdominal distention and the secondary signs of nutritional
deficiency such as weight loss, anaemia and osteomalacia.

Steatorrhoea means an excessive loss of fat in the stools.
They normally contain 5–6 g/day when dietary intake is
70–100 g/day. If fat malabsorption occurs stools can contain
as much as 50–60 g/day.
The causes of malabsorption are divided into groups and are:
  1. Impaired gastric function after gastric surgery and sometimes in atrophic gastritis.

Diarrhoea due to intestinal hurry and bacterial colonisation of the small intestine can both cause malabsorption.

2. Impaired digestion within the intestine.

In pancreatitis and cystic fibrosis, the pancreatic secretion which contains lipase is reduced causing malabsorption of fat. In biliary disease the reduced production of bile salts will prevent fat from being emulsified and cause malabsorption.

3. Impaired small intestinal digestion and absorption.

The final stage of digestion of protein and carbohydrate takes place on the surface of the cells lining the small intestine. If the enzymes are not present there in sufficient quantity, digestion will not be complete and absorption will be impaired. If the lining of the small intestine is abnormal, as in gluten sensitive enteropathy (coeliac disease), or reduced, as in short bowel syndromes, there may not be a sufficient area available for complete absorption to take place. This can be congenital or acquired after the intestine has been damaged. A reduced absorptive surface may be due to surgical resection or mucosal damage, which may be caused by a variety of agents including some drugs. Gluten-sensitive enteropathy is diagnosed in both children and adults. The dietary management of this disorder is explained in Chapter 28.

The principle of dietary treatment of malabsorption involves the exclusion of foods which contain the nutrient that is malabsorbed or causes malabsorption and replacement with suitable alternatives.

For example:

1. Exclude gluten in coeliac disease (see Ch. 28).
2. Exclude the appropriate sugars in disaccharidase deficiency (see Ch. 28).
3. Reduce fat intake in pancreatic insufficiency.
4. If necessary, improve overall nutritional status by providing a suitable high protein, high energy diet with supplements as necessary.

FIBROCYSTIC DISEASE (Cystic fibrosis)

This disorder is usually diagnosed in early childhood. The exocrine glands of the body produce abnormally thick, viscid secretions. All exocrine glands are affected but most clinical problems are due to involvement of the lungs and pancreas. Frequent chest infections result from the congestion of the lungs. Before improved treatment with antibiotics, mucolytic agents and physiotherapy, these were a common cause of death. Pancreatic exocrine insufficiency is present in 80 per cent of cases of cystic fibrosis. The secretions produced by the pancreas block the ducts, eventually causing fibrosis of the gland.

The provision of adequate nutrition in this disorder is essential to ensure and maintain adequate growth and development. Dietary treatment must ensure an adequate intake of all nutrients. This is usually achieved with a high protein, low fat diet, with additional vitamins and oral pancreatic enzyme supplements to aid digestion. The amount of fat tolerated and the amount of enzyme supplement required depend on the severity of the disorder. High energy supplements, such as Hycal and Caloreen, and overnight enteral feeding are sometimes used during periods of infection to overcome the increased metabolic requirements and decreased food intake. In severe cases of pancreatic insufficiency, elemental diets may be used. MCT oil is used to improve the palatability of the low fat diet, to increase its energy content and to aid assimilation.

CHRONIC PANCREATIC EXOCRINE INSUFFICIENCY

This disorder occurs in adults as a result of chronic pancreatitis and is related particularly to alcohol-induced pancreatic damage. Not only is the exocrine function of the pancreas damaged but its endocrine function is often impaired too. This means that diabetes mellitus may be an added complication. The nutritional treatment is a low fat diet with pancreatic enzyme supplements. If diabetes is also present then the type and amount of carbohydrate in the diet will need to be regulated. The amount of fat restriction and enzyme supplementation depends on the residual activity of the pancreas. Only when pancreatic exocrine output is reduced to less than 10 per cent of normal is malabsorption a problem and enzyme supplementation necessary.

Medium chain triglycerides. Most of our dietary fats are

mixtures of long chain triglycerides. These require bile and pancreatic lipase for their digestion and subsequent absorption. Medium chain triglycerides (MCT) do not require bile and lipase for their absorption and are of value when far digestion is impaired. MCT oil is prepared commercially from coconut oil and does not contain all the essential fatty acids. It is added to some low fat diets. MCT oil should be introduced slowly over a period of 7–10 days, mixed with other foods, used in cooking, or added to drinks such as fruit juice, coffee and soup. Care must be taken if it is used for frying because it is easily overheated and then tastes burnt.

Elemental diets (see Ch. 21). These diets contain all the nutrients necessary for complete nutrition in forms that require the minimum of digestion before being absorbed. They were developed originally as low residue diets for the American Space programmes. They have been used for patients with severe disorders of digestive or absorptive function. Their use reduces stool bulk and may enable some degree of bowel rest to be achieved.

HYPOLACTASIA

Congenital alactasia is very rare and is discussed in Chapter 28. However, 70–80 per cent of the non-European population have low lactase levels after childhood (acquired primary hypolactasia). Most of these individuals are free from the symptoms of malabsorption and are not on a strict lactose-free diet. However, if they take large amounts of lactose, such as a large quantity of milk, malabsorption will occur usually resulting in symptoms. This point should be considered when providing high protein supplements and enteral diets based on lactose-containing milk products.

ILEOSTOMY

An ileostomy is fashioned when the colon has been totally removed. If the ileum is normal, nutrients will be absorbed completely there. The water and electrolyte-absorbing capacity of the colon is lost when it is resected. The body rapidly adapts to this and is soon able to maintain water balance. Most ileostomy patients eat a normal diet with the exclusion of a few foods which upsets them by producing flatulence, discomfort or odour. Examples of these foods are onions, peas and cabbage, but these intolerances differ from patient to patient.

Dietary advice

1. A liberal fluid intake is important to prevent water depletion.
2. Avoid foods that cause symptoms.
3. If necessary the ileostomy output at night can be minimised by eating more food in the first half of the day than during the late afternoon and evening.

DISORDERS OF FOOD INTAKE

In serious illnesses, particularly malignant diseases, cachexia is common. Poor appetite and impaired taste result in an inadequate intake of nutrients. Nutritional supplements by the most suitable route will improve the patient's well-being, make nursing easier and prepare the patient better for any necessary procedures.

Clinically, anorexia presents most commonly in the form of anorexia nervosa, which is seen mainly in young women. Anorexics often have a superficial appearance of good health but when the condition persists they become poorly nourished and lose considerable amounts of weight. Anorexia is usually one aspect of a complex personality problem which requires adequate treatment for full recovery. If an adequate dietary intake can be achieved the metabolic and hormonal changes observed are rapidly reversed. Sometimes anorexia may be disguised by self-induced vomiting after an apparently normal meal has ben eaten. These patients occasionally indulge in bulimia, or binge eating of excessive amounts of food.

QUESTIONS

1. Why are patients with peptic ulcer disease advised to eat small frequent meals?
2. What dietary advice would you give to a patient with chronic constipation?
3. High fibre diets are beneficial for diverticular disease and diverticulitis. Why is this?
4. Malabsorption syndrome accompanies many gastrointestinal diseases. List four conditions when dietary treatment is necessary and suggest appropriate dietary changes.

24

Diet in disorders of the liver and biliary system

SUMMARY

The dietary treatment for disorders of the liver and biliary system depend on the individual patient's symptoms.

If fat is not tolerated the diet should be low in fat; the protein intake is reduced when patients are encephalopathic and sodium intake is restricted when ascites is present.

INTRODUCTION

The liver is the largest organ in the body and has many complex functions. These include protein metabolism, carbohydrate storage, the detoxification of some poisons, alcohol metabolism and the production of bile.

Liver injury may be due to the action of infective agents such as the virus of acute infective hepatitis, or to toxic substances such as carbon tetrachloride, chloroform and certain drugs. A feature of the condition is an increased concentration in the blood of the bile pigment bilirubin. The yellow pigmentation which is sometimes observed is known as jaundice and is due to the presence of this pigment in the tissues.

Acute liver injury

Acute liver injury varies greatly in severity, being in some instances so mild that no symptoms are apparent, whereas on the other hand the patient may be seriously ill.

Diet

The patient may be vomiting and nausea and loss of appetite are usually marked. In severe cases it may be necessary to give glucose intravenously to begin with. If fluids can be tolerated by mouth the patient should be encouraged to take as much carbohydrate as possible in the form of fruit drinks with added sugar—300 g or more of glucose or Caloreen may be given daily. Fresh water should be constantly available. With recovery the scope of the diet may be extended in accordance with the appetite of the patient. Formerly a low fat intake was recommended. It has now been shown that fat restriction is unnecessary and that the patient may safely be given whatever foods he fancies. Some patients with acute liver injury have an intolerance of fat, and in this event a low fat diet such as Diet No. 7 is indicated.

HEPATIC CIRRHOSIS

Hepatic cirrhosis is a chronic condition resulting from various forms of liver damage. There may for example be a history of acute infective hepatitis. It is thought that an inadequate food intake may contribute to the development of the cirrhosis which occurs in association with alcoholism. In many cases the cause of the disease remains unknown.

Diet

A balanced diet, adequate in all nutrients, should be given. A protein intake of 1 g/1 kg body weight is sufficient. In certain instances higher protein intake can precipitate encephalopathy. If the patient's appetite is not good, high protein, high energy drinks may be given as supplements.

As the disease progresses the appetite becomes fickle and

there may be associated gastritis; jaundice may be present. It is necessary to exercise special care in the choice of food for these patients and likes and dislikes should be unobtrusively noted. Vitamin supplementation is required. When appetite fails the aim is to provide adequate nourishment in an attractive, easily digested and non-bulky form.

Sodium restriction

Cirrhosis of the liver may be associated with accumulation of fluid in the peritoneal cavity, called ascites, and in this event salt restriction is required. It is important to ensure at the same time that the protein intake is maintained at the required level, and as meat, fish, milk and eggs, which are high in protein content, are relatively high in sodium also, it may be necessary to use a low sodium milk, salt-free bread and unsalted butter in order to achieve an adequate protein intake. Edosol (Cow and Gate) is an example of a low sodium synthetic milk powder which is suitable for the purpose, and if necessary it may be supplemented with a low sodium, protein concentrate such as Casilan. Diet No. 5 is low in sodium and high in protein.

If a *less stringent sodium restriction* is required a minimum of salt may be used in cooking, and fresh milk and ordinary salted bread and butter may be given, with no extra salt added to meals.

DIET NO. 5 Low sodium, high protein diet

Protein, 100 g
Fat, 120 g
Carbohydrate, 300 g   Approximately.
Energy value 11.3 MJ
  (2700 kcal)
Sodium, 500 mg (22 mmol)

Breakfast
Fruit or fruit juice.
Low sodium cereal such as unsalted porridge, Puffed Wheat or Sugar
  Puffs (Quaker Oats Ltd) or Shredded Wheat (Nabisco Foods).
Egg or fish, cooked without salt.
Unsalted bread, with unsalted butter or margarine.
Marmalade or honey.
Tea or coffee with milk from allowance.

Mid-morning
Low sodium, high protein milk drink.

Mid-day meal
Fruit juice.
Average helping unsalted meat or fish.
Unsalted vegetable as desired.
Low sodium sweet such as fruit or jelly with cream, or pastry or
    sponge pudding prepared from low sodium ingredients.
Tea or coffee with milk from allowance.

Tea
Unsalted bread, toasted or made into sandwiches.
Low sodium, high protein milk drink.
Tea with milk from allowance.

Evening meal
Average helping unsalted meat, fish or egg dish.
Unsalted vegetables.
Unsalted bread, with unsalted butter or margarine.
Sweet as at mid-day.
Tea or coffee with milk from allowance.

Bedtime
Low sodium, high protein milk drink.

Milk allowance: 250 ml daily.
Low sodium high protein milk:
Edosol, 500 ml
Casilan, 30 g
Glucose, 50 g
Suggested flavouring—coffee.

Choice of foods

Chapter 22 should be consulted regarding choice of foods,
also suggested seasonings, for low sodium diets.

PORTO-SYSTEMIC ENCEPHALOPATHY

Some patients suffering from liver disease develop signs of
impaired function of the nervous system which may terminate
in coma. The pathogenesis of these is not fully understood,
but they are thought to be due to the presence in the systemic
circulation of poisons which are normally detoxicated by the
liver. It has been found that the presence of nitrogen-

containing material in the intestine plays an important part in precipitating the condition, and one of the measures adopted for its control is a reduction of the protein intake. It is important during this period that the diet should be of sufficient energy value to spare excessive breakdown of tissue protein, and plenty of carbohydrate should be provided in the form of glucose drinks which may be flavoured with fruit juices. If the patient is confused and unco-operative, or in coma, it may be necessary to feed enterally or parenterally. Diet No. 6 (below) provides a protein intake of less than 10 g daily. The protein content of the diet is gradually increased in accordance with the instructions of the physician. Information on the protein content of some average food portions is given on p. 24. This list should be consulted and the necessary adjustments made. In chronic liver disease the level of protein intake at which symptoms recur is noted and the diet restricted accordingly. Diet No. 8 (p. 256) supplies approximately 40 g protein. When patients are discharged from hospital on a low protein diet they must be provided with adequate supplies of the high calorie, low protein products which they took whilst in hospital. If this does not happen the diet will have too low an energy content and be difficult for the patient to manage.

Alcohol

Alcohol now provides a significant proportion of the total energy intake of many people. It is absorbed quickly from the stomach and transported by the hepatic portal vein to the liver where it is metabolised. Alcohol damages the liver tissue of both normal and alcoholic individuals and can cause liver disease. It is excluded from the diets of all patients with liver disease.

DIET NO. 6 Minimum protein diet: sample menu

Protein, not more than 10 g

Breakfast
Sliced orange with sugar.
Protein free bread* with butter and preserves.
Low protein savoury dish such as grilled tomato.
Tea or coffee.

Mid-morning
Coffee, or a fruit drink with added sugar.

Mid-day
Clear vegetable soup with protein free Crispbread* (e.g. Aproten)
One medium potato, with butter and gravy.
Other root or green leafy vegetables as desired.
Canned or stewed fruit with double cream, or a pudding such as
  Apple Crumble made with protein free flour*.
Tea or coffee.

Mid-afternoon
Tea
Protein free biscuits*, or sandwiches such as banana or tomato made
  with protein free bread.

Evening meal
Salad vegetables with oil and vinegar dressing.
or
A cooked vegetable dish such as fried mushrooms, or fried tomato
  and onion, with protein free pasta*.
Protein free bread, toasted or fried.

*For information on proprietary foods especially designed for low
protein diets, see Chapter 25.
Protein free cereal foods may be considered as containing negligible amounts of protein and need not be restricted.

Average helpings: vegetables, with the exception of peas, beans,
lentils and potato.

Unrestricted: fruit, fruit drinks, sugar, glucose, Caloreen, butter,
margarine, and all fats and oils. Liberal use of these will help to
increase the satiety value of the meals and provide an adequate
energy intake.

Coffee-Mate (Carnation Foods Co.) may be added to tea and
coffee.

CHOLECYSTITIS

Cholecystitis, or inflammation of the gall-bladder, is usually
associated with gall-stones. It is frequently accompanied by
obesity and is more common among women than among
men.

Acute cholecystitis

During an acute attack which is not sufficiently severe to
require surgical intervention the dietary treatment is similar

to that employed in the treatment of other acute febrile conditions. The patient should drink plenty of water, and glucose should be given in the form of glucose and fruit drinks.

As the presence of fat in the duodenum stimulates gall-bladder contraction a low fat diet is indicated so that contraction of the gall-bladder is reduced to a minimum during the period of acute inflammation. Skimmed milk is given in preference to full cream milk, and butter, margarine and other fats are withheld. Diet No. 7 below, is suitable for a patient recovering from an acute attack of cholecystitis. Some restriction of carbohydrate is necessary in the event of obesity.

DIET NO. 7 Low fat diet: sample menu

Fat 20 g approximately

Breakfast
Fruit or fruit juice with added sugar, glucose or Caloreen.
Cereal.
Bread, toast or a roll, with marmalade or honey, but without butter.
Tea or coffee.
Skimmed milk and sugar.

Mid-morning
Skimmed milk to drink, with coffee
or
Skimmed milk with Carnation Build-up

Mid-day
Fruit, fruit juice or tomato juice.
Average helping of lean meat or fish, e.g. stewed beef, liver, kidney, poultry, ham, or white fish.
Potato and other vegetables.
Low fat sweet such as jelly and fruit, or a pudding made with skimmed milk
Tea or coffee with skimmed milk and sugar.

Mid-afternoon
Low fat sandwiches e.g. banana, preserves.
or
Water biscuits or Ryvita Crispbread with honey or preserves.

Evening meal
Lean meat or fish as at mid-day.
or
A low fat savoury dish such as baked beans or spaghetti in tomato sauce.
or
Salad vegetables with cottage cheese and pineapple.

Toast or a roll without butter.
Tea or coffee with skimmed milk and sugar.
Fruit with sugar.

Bed-time
Milk drink as at mid-morning

Diets low in fat are correspondingly low in energy value. Provided the patient is not overweight, glucose, sugar and Caloreen should he added to fruit and fruit drinks. Boiled sweets are unrestricted.

Foods to avoid

Whole milk, ice cream, butter, eggs; cheese except cottage cheese
Margarine, lard, and all fats and oils.
Visible fat on meat, and fatty meats such as bacon, tongue, sausages.
Most canned meats e.g. luncheon meat, chopped ham and pork, and corned beef.
Fatty fish such as herring and salmon.
Soups, unless known to be low in fat content.
Pastry, cakes, and most biscuits.
Chocolate, toffee, fudge, nuts, marzipan and lemon curd.

Increase of the fat content

The fat intake may be increased to 40 g daily by the inclusion of 250 ml full cream milk and 15 g butter or margarine.

MCT oil in low fat diets

When fat digestion is impaired, some of the fat of a normal diet may be replaced by MCT oil, the nature and function of which is described in Chapter 10. The energy value and palatability of this diet could be increased by the inclusion of MCT milk shakes, and the frying in MCT oil of items such as bread, potato, mushrooms, tomato and fish.

Chronic cholecystitis

In the case of patients for whom surgery is not advised a suitable long-term regimen is required.

We have seen that the entry of fat into the duodenum is followed by contraction of the gall-bladder and excretion of bile. In the case of patients with chronic cholecystitis, therefore, a normal fat intake helps to counteract atony of the gall-bladder, promotes the drainage of the biliary system and helps to prevent the formation of gall-stones.

Persons with chronic gall-bladder disease frequently suffer from flatulence and epigastric discomfort following meals, and it should be noted that the fats of milk, butter and eggs are better tolerated than the harder types such as dripping, and that fried foods are best avoided. Certain vegetables and fruits may cause flatulence. The idiosyncrasies of the individual patient are the best guide as to which foods should be avoided.

A diet suitable for weight reduction, such as that outlined in Chapter 20, may be necessary if there is associated obesity.

OBSTRUCTIVE JAUNDICE

Obstruction to the flow of bile along the biliary tract may give rise to jaundice, in this case known as obstructive jaundice. Some causes of obstructive jaundice are the presence of gall-stones in the common bile duct and carcinoma of the head of the pancreas. Where possible surgical measures are employed for the relief of the obstruction, but where surgery is not practicable an important aspect of treatment is the provision of a suitable diet.

Since bile is a factor of importance in the digestion of fat, obstructive jaundice is associated with failure of fat digestion and absorption and the excretion of an excessive amount of fat in the faeces. Diarrhoea may also be present. A low fat diet is required and Diet No. 7 may be applied.

Fat intake may be subsequently increased in accordance with the degree of obstruction and the ability of the patient to tolerate fat. It is usually necessary to give the fat-soluble vitamins by intramuscular injection.

QUESTIONS

1. It is important that patients with chronic liver disease have a high-carbohydrate intake.
   Why is this?
   How should the diet be modified to accomplish this?
2. When is a low-fat diet necessary?
3. List six foods excluding butter and margarine which contain fat and should be excluded.

25

Diet in disorders of the kidneys

SUMMARY

The aim of dietary treatment of kidney disease is to ease the task of the kidneys in controlling fluid balance and removing waste products. The protein, sodium and potassium contents of the diet need to be considered. The amount given is reduced if excretion is impaired and increased if abnormal amounts are being lost in the urine.

INTRODUCTION

By excreting a urine of variable composition and volume the kidneys play a major part in maintaining the constant volume and composition of the body fluids. Metabolic waste products are excreted while materials necessary for body function are retained. Renal disease is associated with metabolic disturbances due to impairment of these regulatory activities and in its management modifications of the diet are sometimes employed. In the event of renal failure dietary modifications may be required to play a supporting role, in conjunction with haemodialysis or renal transplant.

ACUTE RENAL FAILURE

A common cause of this condition is circulatory failure due to reduction in blood volume, for example following haemorrhage. It may also result from the action on the renal cells of certain poisons or nephrotoxins, such as mercury or tetrachloride. Renal failure may also occur during the course of acute nephritis, pyelonephritis and other intrinsic diseases of the kidneys.

It is usually characterised by decreased urine flow (oliguria) or cessation of urine flow (anuria), hypertension, and retention of urinary constituents in the blood, or azotaemia, often referred to as uraemia, as a high blood urea level is a prominent feature of this condition. Nausea and vomiting may also be present.

Where possible the immediate cause of the condition is dealt with, e.g. by restoration of blood volume in circulatory failure. Modifications of the diet are directed to delaying as far as possible the accumulation of metabolic end-products requiring excretion by the kidneys, in the hope that normal urine flow will be resumed.

Diet

1. As one of the principal functions of the kidneys is to excrete the products of protein breakdown, protein restriction is required, and a diet supplying 20 g protein of high biological value, and providing all the essential amino acids (essential and non-essential amino acids—refer to p. 20) should be given. The proteins of highest biological value are those of eggs, milk, meat and fish, and these should supply almost all the protein in this diet. As bread and cereal products are normally an important source of protein it is necessary to use specially devised cereal foods, low in protein.

2. It is imperative to ensure an adequate energy intake. This will prevent the utilisation of tissue proteins to meet energy needs.

3. If there is an initial deficit of fluid this is made good. Thereafter the daily allowance should be 400 to 700 ml, plus

an amount equal to the volume of any urine, faeces or vomitus of the previous day.

4. The same applies where sodium and potassium are concerned, any previously incurred deficit being made good. Otherwise intakes of these electrolytes should replace the previous day's loss. In anuria, intakes are reduced to the minimum.

The diet is similar in many respects to the Giordano-Giovanetti diet used for chronic renal failure and Diet No. 9 (p. 257) may be used as a guide, with fluid restriction as described above. It is important to remember that the daily intakes of Hycal and milk must be counted as part of the fluid allowance, and when adapting this diet for acute renal failure it may be necessary to employ some such measure as giving the Hycal undiluted, omitting it altogether, or reducing the milk allowance and giving the equivalent amount of protein in some other form. For example ½ egg is equivalent to 100 ml milk in protein content. If fluid restriction is necessary the dietitian should discuss with the patient how he would like his fluid allocated. For example, some patients find a meal without gravy both unpalatable and unattractive.

Intake of potassium can be adjusted by consulting the list of potassium-containing foods on page 258 and varying the allowance of these as required. If maximum salt restriction is called for, unsalted, low protein bread and unsalted butter should be used, foods should be cooked without salt and none should be added at the table. Obviously salty foods should be avoided. Salt substitutes should not be used without the doctor's permission, because they have a high potassium content.

With salt restriction as detailed above, and including four, 4 mmol portions of fruit or vegetables from the list on page 258, this diet should provide approximately 10 mmol sodium and 25 mmol potassium daily (1 mmol sodium = 23 mg and 1 mmol potassium = 39 mg).

For those patients who cannot be maintained on diet alone dialysis is necessary, and in this case a more liberal diet is given.

If the patient is nauseated to begin with, this symptom may disappear if he can be persuaded to eat all of the diet. Occasionally it is necessary to resort to intravenous feeding for a time.

Diuresis

During diuresis it may be necessary to replace losses of sodium, potassium and fluid. Salts of these minerals are given by mouth. Part of the fluid intake may be given in the form of fruit juices, which have a high potassium content.

For those who do not recover from the acute stage, subsequent dietary management is similar to that of chronic kidney failure as described below.

CHRONIC RENAL FAILURE

Diet plays a major part in the management of this condition. It must be tailored to individual requirements and periodic adjustments are necessary as progressive deterioration takes place.

1. The first essential is an adequate energy intake, sufficient to spare breakdown of body protein.

2. The patient may be excreting excessive quantities of water, sodium and potassium. These losses must be made good and intake is based on output. If the patient is hypertensive and oedematous, salt restriction may be required. Some patients retain potassium to a disproportionate degree and for these potassium restriction, as already outlined on page 254, is indicated.

3. Some reduction of protein intake is necessary and is based on the ability of the kidneys to excrete the nitrogenous material and salts associated with protein metabolism. The patient may tolerate 40 g protein daily to begin with (Diet No. 8, p. 256).

When uraemia has progressed to the stage of producing loss of appetite, nausea and lassitude it is time to consider the 20 g protein diet based on the régime of Giordano and Giovanetti.

Giordano-Giovanetti diet

A diet based on that of Giordano and Giovanetti is given (pp. 257). It will be noted that only 20 g protein are given daily. This is adequate for a limited time provided all the essential amino acids are supplied, and provided the diet is adequate in energy value. Loss of protein in the urine is made good by a corresponding increase in dietary intake.

Varying degrees of salt restriction may be required. For example the omission of salt in cooking and at the table, the avoidance of obviously salty foods including ordinary salted butter, but using the low protein, salted bread, brings the sodium intake to approximately 36 mmol daily.

Appetite may be poor, and great efforts are needed to maintain the energy value of the diet by the use of such high energy, low protein items as sugar, glucose, butter, oils and double cream. Certain foods, including low protein bread and biscuits, are marketed especially for this type of diet. Some of these are listed on page 257.

Supplements of B-complex vitamins and ascorbic acid are required. As this diet is high in carbohydrate, vitamin B$_1$ is particularly important. Iron is sometimes given.

If the patient can be persuaded to eat all of the diet, blood urea will fall, and he will experience a sense of increased comfort and wellbeing which should encourage him to persevere. In some cases the patient may be awaiting acceptance for regular dialysis or for kidney transplantation.

DIET NO. 8 For chronic renal failure
Protein 40 g approximately

Protein intake should be checked by taking a dietary history from the patient at regular intervals.

Take daily

200 ml milk, and in addition,
2 items from the following list—small portion (30 to 50 g) fish or lean meat, 1 egg, average helping (approx. 30 g) cheese provided the diet is not salt-restricted.

The following foods are unrestricted

Bread, biscuits and other cereal foods, butter and all fats and oils. A significant amount of protein is obtained from bread and other baked products. For the purpose of this calculation, intake of these has been estimated as equivalent to 170 g (6 thin slices) bread daily.

Sugar, preserves and confectionery. Tea and coffee. (Some instant coffees have a high potassium content.) Vegetables, fruit and fruit juices provided the diet is not restricted in potassium.

To help ensure adequate energy intake

(a) Take your milk from the 'top of the bottle'.
(b) Add sugar to foods, for example to drinks and stewed fruit.
(c) Take butter and preserves with bread.
(d) Take melted butter or margarine with cooked vegetables; salad oils with salads.
(e) Use frying as a method of cooking where practicable.

DIET NO. 9 Giordano-Giovanetti-Type Diet.
Supplying 20 g protein approximately.

Take daily
200 ml milk.
1 egg, which may be exchanged for 30 g lean meat,* 40 g fish,* or 30 g cheese provided the diet is not salt restricted.
50 g rice boiled in water.
Fruit and vegetables as permitted—the intake of these will vary with potassium requirement. Pulse vegetables should be avoided.

The following items are unrestricted
Low protein bread and biscuits; butter, cooking fats and oils; sugar, glucose and boiled sweets; jam, marmalade and honey.
Caloreen, described in Chapter 16.

Energy intake will vary depending upon the quantities eaten of the unrestricted foods. Estimating intakes of these to be 150 g special bread and biscuit, 60 g butter, 100 g sugar and/or boiled sweets, and 30 g cooking fat or oil, the total energy value of the diet would be around 9.2MJ (2200 kcal) daily.

Flour, bread and biscuits which may be given ad lib.†
Salt free, protein free flour, also protein free bread both salted and unsalted; Welfare Foods (Stockport) Ltd., 63 London Road South, Poynton, Stockport, Cheshire, SK12 1LA.
Aminex low protein biscuits; Distributed by Cow & Gate Baby Foods Ltd., Trowbridge, Wilts.
Aproten low protein flour, semolina, pasta, crispbread and biscuits; Montedison Pharmaceuticals Ltd., Kingmaker House, Station Road, Barnet, Herts., EN5 1NU.
Azeta low protein biscuits; Carlosta Ltd., 33 Ermine Road, London S.E.13.
Juvela protein free mix; Aglutella low protein pasta and semolina; GF Dietary Supplies Ltd., 7 Queensbury Station Parade, Queensbury, Edgware, Middlesex, HA8 5NP.
Low protein biscuits and pastry may be prepared at home using any of the special flours already mentioned, along with fat and sugar. In some areas a suitable bread is prepared locally.

Beverages

Suitable beverages include tea and coffee. It should be noted, however, that some instant coffees have a high potassium content. If maximum restriction of potassium is required both should be weak, and infused for 1 minute only.

Hycal (Beecham Products (UK)) is a suitable fruit flavoured drink, low in electrolyte content. Although high in carbohydrate it is not over-sweet, and is also less likely to cause gastrointestinal side-effects than is a concentrated solution of glucose. It may be diluted with water if preferred. Palatability is increased by chilling. Owing to its high carbohydrate content only approximately 60 per cent is water, requiring consideration if fluids are restricted.

* Weighed after cooking. Some physicians prefer to limited the proteins to those of milk and eggs only, as these are the proteins of highest biological value.

† Each of these items has a small protein content. Details should be sought from the manufacturers.

Table 25.1 The following food portions each contain 4 mmol potassium approximately

beetroot, boiled	40 g
broccoli tops, boiled	150 g
brussels sprouts, boiled	60 g
cabbage, boiled	130 g
carrots, young, boiled	70 g
carrots, old, boiled	180 g
cauliflower, boiled	100 g
celery, raw	60 g
celery, boiled	120 g
cucumber	110 g
french beans, boiled	150 g
leek, boiled	60 g
lettuce	80 g
mushrooms, fried	30 g
onion, boiled	200 g
onion, fried	60 g
onion, spring, raw	70 g
parsnip, boiled	50 g
potato, boiled	50 g
swede, boiled	150 g
tomato, raw	50 g
turnip, boiled	100 g
vegetable marrow, boiled	190 g
apples, raw, weighed with skin & core	180 g
apricots, canned, fruit & syrup weighed	60 g
banana, weighed with skin	80 g
grapefruit, without skin	70 g
grapes	60 g

mandarins, canned, fruit and syrup weighed	160 g
melon, cantaloupe, flesh only	50 g
melon, yellow, flesh only	70 g
olives in brine, weighed with stones	200 g
orange, weighed without peel	80 g
orange juice	90 ml
peaches, fresh, weighed with stones	70 g
peaches, canned, fruit and syrup weighed	100 g
pears, weighed with skin and core	170 g
pears, canned, fruit and syrup weighed	170 g
plums, victoria dessert, weighed with stones	90 g
prunes, dried, raw, weighed with stones	20 g
raspberries	70 g
rhubarb, raw	40 g
strawberries	100 g

THE NEPHROTIC SYNDROME

This disease runs a protracted course, with a fatal outcome in a proportion of cases. The prognosis is much more favourable for children than for adults. The principal features are loss of protein, especially albumin, in the urine, a decrease in the plasma albumin level, marked oedema, and the absence of uraemia until a late stage of the illness.

Principles of dietary treatment

1. Protein intake should be high to compensate for urinary loss and prevent depletion of body tissue. At least 100 g protein should be given daily. There are no contraindications to a high protein diet in the initial stages of this form of kidney disease as the ability of the kidneys to excrete metabolic waste products is unimpaired.

2. A restriction of the sodium intake may be necessary to help to counteract the oedema which follows the fall in plasma albumin level.

Administration of the diet

Diet No. 5 may be used as a basis when constructing diets for patients with the nephrotic syndrome. In most cases a moderate salt restriction, or no-added-salt type of diet will suffice.

QUESTIONS

1. List:
   a. Four foods which are high in energy but low in protein
   b. Four foods with both a high protein and a high sodium content
   c. Four foods with a high potassium content.
2. When protein intake is restricted, why should the protein-containing foods have a high biological value? Which protein containing foods have a high biological value?
3. What dietary restrictions would you expect to see imposed on a patient with acute renal failure?

26

Diet in diabetes mellitus

SUMMARY

Diabetes is due to an inadequate supply of insulin. Dietary treatment is a necessary part of the management of all diabetics and often includes weight reduction.

All nutrients are important in the diabetic diet. Carbohydrate-containing foods are distributed throughout the day to balance the available insulin. There are two diet types: the sugar-free diet and the carbohydrate-exchange diet. The type of diet prescribed for a diabetic depends on the severity of the diabetes, the type of treatment and his lifestyle.

INTRODUCTION

Diabetes mellitus occurs when the amount of insulin produced is insufficient for normal metabolism. The islet cells of the pancreas produce the hormones insulin and glucagon (p. 9), which are both involved in the regulation of blood glucose concentration. In the past, most emphasis has been placed on the disordered carbohydrate metabolism occurring in diabetes mellitus. This was because glucose in the urine and blood could be measured easily.

Insulin is secreted in response to an increase in the blood glucose. Then, as the blood glucose drops, so does the amount of insulin produced, and the secreted insulin in the bloodstream is metabolised. Insulin has three major sites of action: muscle, liver and adipose tissue. It has a large number of actions at these sites, the most important of which are listed below.

Effects of insulin on muscle

Increases glucose entry into the muscle cells.
Increases protein synthesis.
Increases glycogen synthesis.
Decreases protein breakdown.

Effects of insulin on liver

Increases protein synthesis.
Increases lipid synthesis.
Increases glycogen synthesis.
Decreases the production of glucose from amino acids.

Effects of insulin on adipose tissue

Increases glucose entry into the fat cells.
Increases lipid synthesis.

From this list it can be seen that lack of insulin leads not only to disordered carbohydrate metabolism but also to disordered protein and fat metabolism.

Blood glucose

The amount of glucose in the blood depends on the balance between the amounts entering and leaving it. Glucose entering the blood comes from three sources:

1. Carbohydrate containing foods. Once digested and absorbed these are the body's most important glucose source.

2. Glycogen. This is stored in the muscle and liver and is broken down to release glucose.

3. *Some amino acids* are broken down by the liver to produce glucose.

Insulin is *not* needed for any of these processes to occur. Once glucose has entered the bloodstream, insulin *is* needed to enable glucose to leave the blood and enter the tissues. In the non-diabetic person, glucose leaving the circulation is used in two ways:

1. *immediate energy* for all tissues;
2. *stored energy* as glycogen in liver and muscle, and fat in the adipose tissue.

The blood glucose responses to a glucose tolerance test

A standard glucose tolerance test now consists of 75 g glucose in 250 ml water. The blood glucose responses of a non-diabetic and a diabetic can be seen in Figure 26.1.

The normal fasting blood glucose range is 3–5 mmol/l which rises to a maximum of 8 mmol/l within the first hour after swallowing the glucose. The rise in blood glucose is modified by the action of insulin produced in response to the increase in blood glucose. By the end of $2\frac{1}{2}$ hours the blood glucose has returned to the fasting value.

In the diabetic the lack of insulin will mean that glucose cannot leave the circulation. Consequently, the blood glucose rises to a higher peak and the return to the fasting value takes longer. The fasting level in diabetics is higher than in non-diabetics.

In the kidney, glucose passes freely into the glomerular filtrate but is normally reabsorbed before it leaves the renal tubule thus preventing the loss of glucose in the urine. When the blood glucose rises above the renal threshold (about 10 mmol/l), the kidney can no longer resorb all the glucose and some is lost in the urine.

Symptoms of diabetes mellitus

Glycosuria due to a high blood glucose is accompanied by an increased loss of water and electrolytes. This osmotic diuresis leads to increased thirst, dehydration, electrolyte disturbances and weight loss. To compensate for the unavailability of glucose as an energy source, the body increases the rates at

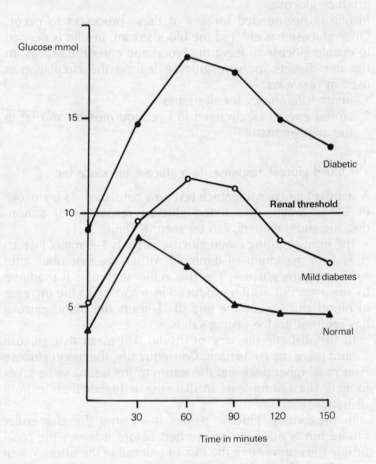

Figure 26.1 Blood glucose response to glucose tolerance test.

which glycogen and fat are broken down to release energy sources, and produces glucose from the breakdown of body protein. This leads to the production of ketones and ketoacids which are toxic. These metabolic disturbances eventually lead to diabetic coma if untreated.

From the point of view of treatment, diabetics fall into two groups:

	Age of onset	Incidence	Treatment
Type 1 Insulin dependent	Under 30 yrs often in childhood	2 in 1000 (below age of 20)	Insulin and diet
Type 2 Non-insulin dependent	Middle and old age	5–10 in 1000	Oral hypoglycaemic drugs and diet, or diet only

Figure 26.2 illustrates the methods of treating diabetics.

All diabetics need dietary advice

1. Diabetics who do not require insulin injections need dietary advice to ensure efficient use of their available insulin.
2. Diabetics who require insulin injections need dietary advice to ensure that the timing of their meals and the carbohydrate content coincides with the activity of the injected insulin.
3. Obese diabetics need to be advised on how to lose weight.

Aims of dietary treatment

1. To restore and maintain the blood glucose to within the normal range, so preventing glycosuria and its associated symptoms.

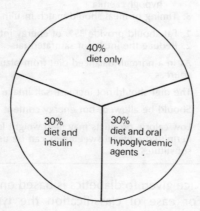

Figure 26.2 How diabetics are treated.

2. To reduce the size of post-prandial blood glucose swings. This, together with the normalisation of blood glucose, helps to prevent the development of the late complications including microvascular disease.
3. To provide an adequate supply of all nutrients—allowing normal growth and tissue repair.
4. To restore and maintain normal body weight.

For centuries diets for diabetics have been surrounded by controversy and confusion. Before the discovery of insulin, when diet was the only treatment for diabetes, success was claimed for a variety of obscure diets. These included diets based on rice and on rancid meat. In 1982, the British Diabetic Association assessed the diets prescribed for diabetics and the evidence for their success. As a result of this they published new recommendations for diabetic diets. The recommendations are summarised in Table 26.1.

Table 26.1 Recommendations for diabetic diets

Nutrient	Recommendations
Energy (total kcals)	1. a. Restrict for obese diabetics b. Must not exceed requirements for normal weight diabetic 2. At least half the energy intake should be as carbohydrate
Carbohydrate	1. Encourage the use of fibre-rich unrefined foods 2. a. Should be as polysaccharides rather than simple sugars b. Sugars should only be used during illness and for hypoglycaemia 3. Timing of meal should match insulin activity
Fat	1. Fat should provide 35% of energy intake at most 2. Reduce the intake of saturated fats
Protein	As in a normal, balanced diet from plant and animal sources
Salt	The diet should not increase salt intake
Alcohol	Should be allowed, but energy content remembered
Special products	Low calorie products may help weight loss Permitted artificial sweeteners can be used as sugar substitutes

The dietary advice given to diabetics is based on these recommendations. For ease of classification the type of dietary advice given is divided into three types; whether the diet is based on one or more of these types depends on the severity of the diabetes, type of treatment, personality, age, weight and lifestyle of the diabetic.

The three types are:

1. Weight reduction followed by weight maintenance.
2. Sugar-free.
3. Carbohydrate-exchange system.

1. Weight-reducing diets

The first priority in treating the obese diabetic is weight loss. The diabetic on a reducing diet must appreciate the need to lose weight and that weight once lost must never be regained. There are many different diets for weight reduction (see Ch. 6). If the diabetes is mild, any reducing diet is suitable if it is nutritionally adequate and provides the basis for a subsequent weight maintenance diet. Initially, overweight diabetics are well motivated and keen to lose weight. This must be capitalised on and encouraged by regular weight checks. Some diabetics benefit from the support and pressures of a slimming group and that must be encouraged.

2. Sugar-free diet

This type of diet is used for elderly diabetics who do not need insulin injections. It is based on two principles:

a. Exclusion of sugar and sugar-containing foods.
b. Regular consumption of carbohydrate containing foods as part of all meals.

Sugar and sugar-containing foods are excluded because they are digested and absorbed quickly and so cause a rapid rise in the blood glucose. These foods are:

    All types of sugar

    Honey, jam and marmalade

    Sweets and chocolates

    Cream, jam and chocolate biscuits

    Cakes and puddings

    Tinned fruit in syrup

    Fruit squashes and fizzy drinks that contain sugar.

Each meal must contain carbohydrate in the form of starch and must be regularly spaced throughout the day. The amount of carbohydrate allowed for each meal depends on the total energy requirement of the individual. Providing the carbohydrate as starch and distributing it evenly throughout the day will achieve the best match between carbohydrate intake and the available insulin.

Diet plan for a diabetic treated by diet alone

Mrs Smith is a 75-year-old widow who lives by herself. She is not overweight and is able to prepare her own meals. Her diabetes was diagnosed five years ago and is treated by diet alone. On Tuesdays and Thursdays she has lunch at a local authority lunch club. On Fridays her daughter comes to see her, bringing lunch from the local fish and chip shop with her.

DIET NO. 10
Mrs Smith's diet

Breakfast		Tea
		Fruit juice
		2 Weetabix and milk
		1 slice wholemeal toast and butter
Mid-morning		Coffee and 1 biscuit
Lunch	Lunch Club	Fridays	Rest of week
	Meat	Fried fish	Meat or fish
	Vegetable	(no batter)	Vegetable
	1 potato	2 slices bread	2 potatoes
	Unsweetened	with butter	Fresh or stewed
	milk pudding	1 apple	fruit
Mid-afternoon		Tea
Supper		2 slices bread and butter
		Egg or cheese
		Salad or fresh fruit
Bedtime		2 plain biscuits and tea

---

3. The carbohydrate exchange system

This is designed to provide a method of regulating the carbohydrate precisely. It is used both for those diabetics who are treated with insulin injections and those on high doses of hypoglycaemic agents. A diet based on this system is more complicated for the diabetic to manage, but has the advantage of providing a diet which is more flexible and varied than the sugar-free type.

Carbohydrate exchanges—what are they?

In this country it is conventional for a carbohydrate exchange to be the amount of food which on chemical analysis contains 10 g of carbohydrate. A list of these carbohydrate exchanges has been produced by the British Diabetic Association. All diabetics and dietitians must use this standard list. The interchange of exchanges in the diet enables the diabetic to include a variety of foods in a meal and keep the carbohydrate content constant. Examples of 10 g exchanges are on page 271.

How many exchanges?

The number of carbohydrate exchanges a diabetic is allowed in a day depends on two factors:
1. His total energy requirement
2. The percentage of the total energy requirement that is to be provided by carbohydrate.

The total energy requirement is decided after the diabetic's current diet has been assessed. It is usual to aim for 55 per cent of the total energy to be provided by carbohydrate.

There is a wide variation in the number of carbohydrate exchanges allowed. For example, an overweight diabetic may only be allowed 12 (120 g carbohydrate) a day while an 'ideal weight' diabetic is allowed 30 (300 g carbohydrate) a day. Of course, both of these diabetics have different total energy requirements.

When are they eaten?

The way in which the carbohydrate exchanges are distributed depends on the type of treatment the diabetic is receiving. The aim is to balance insulin activity with food and so prevent both hypo- and hyperglycaemia.

Diabetics who are treated with slow-acting insulin or oral hypoglycaemic agents have their carbohydrate allocated evenly throughout the day. However, if treatment is with mixtures of insulin or fast-acting insulins, then most of the carbohydrate should be eaten at the times of peak insulin activity.

Examples

The charts below show the daily distribution of carbohydrate as exchanges for two diabetics who have the same daily carbohydrate allowance but different insulin regimes.

Mr Jones injects lente insulin before breakfast.

Mr Brown injects actrapid insulin before breakfast and supper.

Mr Jones	Breakfast	Mid-morning	Lunch	Mid-afternoon	Supper	Bedtime
Number of exchanges	4	2	5	2	5	2
Lente injection ↑						

Mr Brown	6	1	4	1	6	2
Actrapid injections ↑			↑			

Which carbohydrate is best?

Exchange lists include a wide variety of foods from pitta bread to pomegranites.However, good diabetic control is only obtained if they are used sensibly. The rises in blood glucose after different carbohydrate exchanges are not the same. This means that diabetics need to be told both how many exchanges they are allowed for a meal and the most suitable type of exchanges for that meal.

The example in Table 26.2 shows what one diabetic's diet, based on the carbohydrate exchange system, means when it is considered as a day's menu. The right hand column shows how the 250 g carbohydrate is allocated to meals.

Christopher is 22 years old and lives with his parents. He has two injections of actrapid, one before breakfast and the other before supper. He is allowed 250 g carbohydrate a day.

The importance of dietary fibre in the diabetic diet

The use of dietary fibre supplements as a treatment for diabetes had already been mentioned in Chapter 8. Unrefined high fibre foods are beneficial to diabetics for three reasons:

Table 26.2 Diet plan for a patient treated with insulin and a carbohydrate-exchange diet

Meal	Carbohydrate allowance	Amount of food	Carbohydrate content	Number of exchanges	Total exchanges
Breakfast (Insulin injected)	70	½ glass orange juice	10	1	
		2 Weetabix	20	2	
		1 cup milk	10	1	
		3 slices wholemeal toast	30	3	7
Mid-morning	20	Coffee			
		1 apple	10	1	
		2 plain biscuits	10	1	2
Lunch	50	Sandwiches made from 4 slices			
		wholemeal bread	40	4	
		1 orange	10	1	5
Mid-afternoon	10	Tea			
		2 biscuits	10	1	1
Supper (Insulin injected)	80	Meat			
		Portion of peas	10	1	
		4 boiled potatoes	40	4	
		Wholemeal apple crumble	20	2	
		Custard	10	1	8
Bed time	20	Tea			
		2 slices wholemeal bread as a			
		sandwich	20	2	2
Total	250		250	25	25

All bread from a small wholemeal loaf spread with margarine high in polyunsaturates
All tea and coffee with a small amount of milk

1. Like the rest of the population, diabetics need fibre in the diet for healthy functioning of the gastrointestinal tract.

2. Carbohydrate contained in foods that are rich in the viscous types of fibre is absorbed slowly, producing a lower rise in the blood glucose. An example of this type of food is the lentil.

3. The unrefined fibre-rich form of a food is more bulky and takes longer to eat than its fibre-depleted counterpart. For example, it takes 12 times as long to eat apples as it does to drink the same amount of carbohydrate in apple juice. For the obese diabetic whose total energy intake is restricted, the extra bulk and feeling of satiety after eating the fibre-rich food is of particular value.

Protein and fat in the diabetic diet

Diabetics are advised to keep the proportion of their total energy intake that comes from fat to 35 per cent or less. By reducing total fat and saturated fat intake and increasing the amount of polyunsaturated fat in the diet, it is hoped to reduce the risk of arterial disease. This is in keeping with the recommendations of a healthy diet for the rest of the population (see Ch. 12). Fat intake can be controlled by the following rules.

1. Avoid fried and fatty foods.
2. Eat full cream cheese in moderation.

Some diabetics, but not all, will also be advised to use skimmed milk and polyunsaturated margarine instead of full cream milk and butter.

Protein is an important nutrient. A well planned balanced diet contains proteins from a variety of sources, both animal and plant.

Special dietary foods for diabetics

Chemists and health food shops are full of products which are made especially for diabetics or are labelled suitable for diabetics. Expensive mistakes can be avoided if diabetics know which types of product are suitable for them and which are not. The special products can be divided into three groups.

1. Low calorie sugar-free products

Fruit tinned in water or unsweetened fruit juice
Low calorie soups
Sugar-free fruit squashes and carbonated drinks

All diabetics including the overweight will find these useful. However, the calorie content of the fruits and soups is not negligible and must be counted.

2. Special diabetic products

These are luxury items and include:
Diabetic cakes and biscuits
Diabetic sweets and chocolates
Diabetic preserves

These products are sucrose-free and the alternative sweetening agents used are fructose and sorbitol. They are high in calories, often containing more calories than the ordinary products, and so are unsuitable for the overweight. They are also expensive. It is better to exclude sugar-containing foods or restrict them than to replace them with these special foods.

Diabetic lager has a lower carbohydrate content than ordinary lager. The carbohydrate is replaced with alcohol making the lager higher in calories and more intoxicating!

Artificial sweeteners

Three sweetening alternatives to sugar are available in this country. They are saccharine, sorbitol and fructose.

Saccharine is the only calorie-free sweetener. It is used in some reducing diets and can be added to drinks and cooked food. If it is added to food before it is cooked it gives a metallic taste. The British Diabetic Association advise that no more than 14 saccharine tablets should be taked a day. This may be an unnecessarily harsh restriction because there is doubt over the evidence for saccharine toxicity in the amounts normally taken by diabetics.

The cost of the diabetic diet

A diabetic should not need to spend more on food when he

is on a diet unless his previous diet was particularly poor or peculiar. Those who find the diet expensive are usually the diabetics who are buying expensive diabetic products or large amounts of fresh fruit and vegetables out of season.

A special dietary allowance is payable to diabetics who receive Supplementary Benefit. See Supplementary Benefit Information Leaflet SB8.

The diabetic diet and exercise

During exercise the entry of glucose into muscle increases. This increase also occurs in the absence of insulin. As a result of this the blood glucose concentration drops. To compensate for this drop and prevent hypoglycaemia diabetics need extra carbohydrate (10–20 g) before exercise. It is not necessary to subtract this carbohydrate from the next meal's allowance, it is an addition needed for the additional exercise. This allowance is popular with children who are allowed extra carbohydrate as sweets before swimming, games or a fight!

Hypoglycaemia

Hypoglycaemia can occur in diabetics who are treated by insulin and long-acting oral hypoglycaemic drugs. The causes of a low blood sugar include:

>Increased energy expenditure such as extra or unexpected activity
>Delayed meal
>Lack of carbohydrate at a meal
>Mismeasurement of the insulin dose.

The diabetic is usually aware of the symptoms of hypoglycaemia in himself. If he experiences these symptoms he should take three sugar lumps (=15 g carbohydrate) and repeat this in ten minute intervals, if necessary. Diabetics should always carry some sugar with them for this reason

Diet in illness

When unwell, diabetics must continue to take their hypoglycaemic agents and inject their insulin to ensure normal metabolism. This means that they must eat enough carbohydrate to balance the insulin activity even though they may not feel hungry. Carbohydrate exchanges that are easily eaten and quickly prepared should be used. Examples of these exhanges are tinned soup, milk drinks, ice cream, yoghurt and fruit juice.

Example

Janice is a 19-year-old secretary who normally eats lunch in the canteen at work. Her lunch time carbohydrate allowance is 50 g which is provided by
  1 exchange fruit juice
  3 exchanges potato
  1 exchange as fruit
When she has 'flu and stays at home her 50 g carbohydrate is provided by
  1 exchange fruit juice
  2 exchanges tinned soup
  2 exchanges fruit yoghurt

THE BRITISH DIABETIC ASSOCIATION

10 Queen Anne Street
London WIM OB6

Diabetics should join the Association as its local branch meetings provide a link between diabetics. The literature published by the Association gives practical advice about a wide variety of topics.

QUESTIONS

1. How does insulin affect carbohydrate metabolism?
2. What are the most usual sources of carbohydrate in the diet?
3. What is a carbohydrate exchange?
4. List five 10 g carbohydrate exchanges.
5. What causes glycosuria?

27

Diet and anaemia; allergic conditions; some food and drug interactions

SUMMARY

Diet and anaemia

Dietary factors known to be essential for the normal synthesis of red blood cells are iron, vitamin B_{12}, folic acid, ascorbic acid and protein. Deficiency of any one of these interferes with the formation of red blood cells and leads to the development of anaemia. Of the various types, that due to lack of iron is by far the most common.

Food allergies

Most foods are suspected of causing an allergic response in someone. Foods commonly listed include shell fish, eggs, milk and strawberries. It is essential that a suspected food allergy is properly investigated before a restricted diet is adopted.

Iron deficiency anaemia

Iron deficiency anaemia is of widespread occurrence, not only in the United Kingdom but throughout the world. It is due to a lack of iron for the formation of haemoglobin, the oxygen-carrying pigment of the red cells of the blood. An insufficiency of this mineral gives rise to a reduction in the number and size of the red blood corpuscles and in their content of haemoglobin. The person becomes pale, and is weak and easily tired. Various factors contribute to bring about this condition.

1. The diet may be low in iron.

2. Requirement may be increased due to loss of blood, for instance as a result of injury, from a peptic ulcer or haemorrhoids, or as a result of nose-bleeding, or excessive menstrual loss.

3. Absorption of iron may be impaired, as occurs in certain disorders of the alimentary tract.

Sometimes several factors are involved.

Iron deficiency anaemia occurs commonly among women, especially those with large menstrual losses or who have had repeated pregnancies, and among children and adolescents, whose iron requirements are high because growth is taking place. Infants are liable to develop anaemia, especially if kept for a long time on a milk diet without adequate supplements, as both human and cow's milk are poor sources of iron. In this country, the incidence of iron deficiency anaemia has been reduced by better medical care and living standards. Surveys of populations in Western Europe show that the incidence of iron deficiency anaemia amongst women of child-bearing age to be between 15 and 25 per cent. Another group who are likely to suffer from anaemia are the over-75 age group, particularly those who have difficulty chewing food.

Treatment and prevention

As this mineral is present in foods in comparatively small amounts, the most effective way to correct iron deficiency anaemia once it has become established is to administer iron in medicinal form. Treatment must also be given for any underlying condition which may be present, such as haemorrhoids.

If faulty eating habits have played a part in bringing about the anaemia these must be corrected in order to prevent a recurrence of the condition and the patient should be shown how to select a good mixed diet. Children, adolescents and pregnant and nursing women should take at least one egg every day and liver once weekly. Certain individuals, for example those who suffer from unavoidable chronic blood loss, or who have had repeated pregnancies, may require a daily maintenance dose of medicinal iron to prevent the development of anaemia. The occurrence of iron deficiency anaemia in infancy may be largely prevented (*a*) by ensuring that the mother has an adequate intake of iron during pregnancy, so that the needs of the fetus are fully met, and (*b*) by giving the infant supplementary foods of high iron content, such as egg yolk, scraped liver and other meats, and fortified infant cereal foods, at the end of the fourth month.

Vitamin B$_{12}$

Lack of vitamin B$_{12}$, giving rise to pernicious anaemia, is the result of failure to absorb the vitamin from the alimentary tract. Because the lack of intrinsic factor means that vitamin B$_{12}$ cannot be absorbed, this condition cannot be cured or prevented by a diet rich in vitamin B$_{12}$ or oral vitamin supplements. Injections are necessary instead. Dietary deficiency of vitamin B$_{12}$ occurs, in the presence of normal absorption, only in Vegans who eat no animals products at all.

Folic acid

Dietary deficiency of folic acid is thought to play a part in bringing about the megaloblastic anaemia which occasionally occurs in pregnancy. In this country it is also seen in premature infancts and the elderly. Dietary deficiency of folic acid is frequently observed among pregnant women in tropical countries.

Further information of these vitamins is given in Chapter 6.

Ascorbic acid

Anaemia due to lack of ascorbic acid is sometimes found in conjunction with scurvy.

Protein

A serious deficiency of protein, as encountered in some tropical and subtropical countries (p. 26), may result in lack of protein for the structure of the red blood corpuscles and contribute to the development of anaemia.

FOOD ALLERGIES

The term allergy is used to describe an immunological reaction on the part of the body to an agent which does not normally give rise to a reaction. The material which brings about the reaction is known as the allergen. Foods liable to cause such a reaction include milk, eggs, cereals, shellfish and certain fruits. Tartrazine, a colouring agent used in food, can cause allergic reactions. Examples of reactions which occur are asthma, hayfever, urticaria and skin rashes, abdominal symptoms, and in severe cases, anaphylactic shock.

In the case of food allergies, if the allergen can be identified it can then be eliminated from the diet. Sometimes the reaction is so immediate and the conclusion so obvious that identification does not present a problem. In doubtful cases, the occurrence of symptoms following ingestion of the suspected food on three separate occasions will help to establish the diagnosis.

In difficult cases and where several foods are suspected, elimination diets are sometimes employed. The patient is given a list of foods unlikely to cause a reaction and told to eat only these for a specified number of days. Foods are then introduced at intervals, one at a time, and by this means allergens may sometimes be identified. Skin sensitivity tests may also be helpful in making a diagnosis.

The specialised assistance of a dietitian is necessary for both diagnosis and treatment of food allergies. Some of the items known to cause allergies are present, often in small but nevertheless significant amounts, in many foods in which their presence is totally unsuspected, being added for purely technical reasons. Elimination diets are necessarily unbalanced and require expert supervision. Finally, when a diagnosis has been made it is necessary to have expert advice on all the possible dietary sources of the allergens identified. Some of these dietary sources may be far from obvious.

After some months, a person may develop a tolerance of the food to which they had been previously allergic. A tentative trial can be made of the food in question; however, all such experimentation should be strictly supervised by a physician.

SOME FOOD AND DRUG INTERACTIONS

Professor A. H. G. Love, Queen's University, Belfast

It is well recognised that the clinical response to drug administration varies widely between individuals. When drugs are taken by mouth the time of onset, the duration and the intensity of drug action are determined partly by the characteristics of absorption from the gastrointestinal tract.

Drug absorption is delayed by the presence of food in the stomach. Thus the consumption of antibiotics after a meal leads to much lower blood concentrations than when the drugs are taken on an empty stomach. This could clearly render such treatment ineffective if the plasma and tissue concentrations are reduced below the minimal needed to inhibit bacterial growth.

Certain chemical substances and even certain foods in the intestine have a specific inhibitory effect on absorption. Thus eggs have been shown to reduce iron absorption, various salts of calcium, magnesium, iron and aluminium (present in antacids and saline purgatives) interfere with absorption of tetracyclines.

Substances which interfere with absorption of fat and of fat-soluble vitamins such as liquid paraffin and cholestyramine (Questran) may also influence drug action. Chronic consumption of these agents can lead to a relative deficiency of vitamin K. Drugs which alter the intestinal flora by an antibacterial action can indirectly influence absorption of drugs and availability of nutrients. Much has been made of the effect of tetracyclines on absorption of B vitamins but it is unlikely that the influence is strong. Relative deficiency of vitamin K is produced by gut sterilisation with neomycin so that anticoagulants have enhanced action.

It has been established that long-term treatment of epilepsy with certain anticonvulsants, notably phenytoin sodium, results in an increased folate requirement with the possible development of megaloblastic anaemia. This group of drugs can also lead to calcium unavailability with the induction of rickets or osteomalacia. This is also a potential hazard of high fibre diets because of their phytate content

Perhaps one of the most important food-drug interactions is exemplified by a group of drugs, monoamine oxidase inhibitors (MAO inhibitors), used in the treatment of depression. Monoamine oxidase is one of the enzymes responsible for the breakdown of tissue adrenaline, noradrenaline and serotonin. Noradrenaline is particularly important since it leaves the circulation and is stored at nerve endings. If a patient is receiving MAO inhibitors greater quantities of noradrenaline are stored because it is not broken down to inactive forms. If such a patient ingests tyramine then this stored noradrenaline is released and may produce a fatal rise in blood pressure. Foods which contain tyramine in large quantities and should therefore be avoided are:

All hard cheeses, processed cheeses and cheese spreads; cottage cheese and cream cheese are safe;

Meat or yeast extracts such as Marmite and Bovril. Alcoholic drinks other than in true moderation. Problems may arise with any alcoholic beverage but particularly high tyramine values are found in red Chianti type wines; broad bean pods and the skins of bananas; pickled herrings.

Avoid foods that have previously produced unpleasant symptoms.

Eat only fresh food, or freshly prepared foods that have been frozen or canned. This applies particularly to meat, fish, poultry, game and offal.

Avoid foods eaten in the fermented state.

Anyone giving dietary advice to patients receiving these drugs should refer to Adverse Drug Reaction Bulletin No. 58, June 1976, for more detailed information on the application of these restrictions.

28

Diet in some disorders encountered in paediatrics

SUMMARY

These diets are based on the same principles:
1. The exclusion or limiting of foods which contain nutrients which cannot be absorbed, cannot be metabolised, or are harmful.
2. The provision of a diet which provides an adequate intake of all essential nutrients, ensuring that the child can grow and develop normally.

GLUTEN SENSITIVE ENTEROPATHY (Coeliac disease)

Coeliac disease occurs primarily in early childhood and is characterised by inadequate absorption of food. Structural changes occur in the mucosa of the small bowel. Symptoms of the disease include loss of appetite, wasting, flatulence and abdominal distension. Impaired fat absorption gives rise to an increased excretion of fat in the faeces which are loose, pale in colour and foul-smelling. Anaemia is usually present.

The disturbance is due to the effect on certain susceptible individuals of the protein gluten as it occurs in wheat and rye flours. Gluten is in fact a mixture of two proteins, glutenin and gliadin. Gliadin is the fraction which gives rise to coeliac disease. The mechanism of action of gliadin in bringing about its harmful effect is not yet fully understood.

Diet

The treatment consists in providing a diet completely free from the gluten of wheat or rye. Some hospitals also exclude oats. This is a regimen requiring great vigilance as wheat flour is used in the preparation of a very large variety of foods. In Table 28.1 are listed some foods which may, and some which may not be included in a gluten free diet. In some cases foods generally regarded as being unsuitable are available in a gluten free form.

A gluten free but otherwise normal diet is embarked upon straight away. Vitamin supplementation may be necessary and anaemia is treated by administration of iron. Occasionally the child may be very ill and miserable and the nurse must be prepared to exercise much patience and ingenuity in overcoming a disinclination for food. Following initiation of the diet, improvement is usually marked, and this helps to motivate the parents and impress them with the necessity for continuing with it.

In very ill children damage to the intestinal mucosa may be such that digestion of disaccharides is impaired—notably digestion of lactose (milk sugar). In this event the diet should be free from milk in the early stages of treatment. Occasionally a multiple malabsorption state is encountered involving the disaccharides, protein and fat. Some proprietary foods useful in the treatment of multiple malabsorption states are listed later in this chapter.

Prognosis

If a gluten free dietary regimen is consistently maintained normal health and development can be expected. The mother must understand that occasional lapses, although apparently trivial, will impair the beneficial effects of the diet. It is generally accepted that for optimum benefit a gluten free diet must be maintained for life.

Proprietary cereal foods designed for the treatment of

Table 28.1 Classification of foods for a diet free from wheat or rye gluten

Foods not allowed	Foods allowed
Bread, biscuits, cakes or puddings which contain ordinary flour. Proprietary cake and pudding · mixes. Bought baking powders. Starch-reduced foods, including Energen Rolls. Semolina, farola, macaroni, spaghetti, vermicelli, Shredded Wheat, Weetabix, Puffed Wheat, Vita-Weat, Ryvita, Bemax, proprietary infant cereal foods.	Bread, biscuits, cakes, etc., made from gluten free flour substitute Yeast, or a gluten free chemical raising agent, may be used for leavening. Rice, ground rice, sago, tapioca, oatmeal, pure cornflour. Custard powders prepared from cornflour. Kellogg's Cornflakes and Rice Krispies
Vegetables canned in sauce.	All fresh, frozen or dried vegetables, and vegetables canned in brine. All fruits—fresh, frozen, canned or dried.
Canned and packed soups.	Home-made soups which may be thickened with lentils, split peas, gluten free flour, or a suitable cereal such as rice.
Canned meats, canned fish in sauce, fish coated with batter or crumbs, fish and meat pastes, sausages, prepared gravy mixtures.	All freshly cooked meat and fish. Gravy may be thickened with cornflour, Bovril or Marmite may be added if desired.
Cheese spreads of uncertain composition.	Milk, eggs, cheese. Butter, margarine, dripping and all fats.
Horlick's Malted Milk and Benger's Food	Cocoa, Ovaltine, coffee, tea, minerals, fruit juices.
Salad creams, bottled sauces, pickles in sauce, commercial chutneys.	Vinegar, salt, flavouring essences and herbs, pickles in clear vinegar. Pepper and spices.
All sweets, chocolates and ice cream of unknown composition. Commercially prepared lemon curd.	Jam, marmalade, sugar, glucose, treacle, syrup, clear boiled sweets, jellies.

coeliac disease are available. They include flour, bread, biscuits and pasta. The majority of them can be prescribed by a doctor. Some firms marketing these are listed below.

Cow and Gate Baby Foods, P.O. Box 99, Trowbridge, Wilts., BA14 8HZ.
Farley Health Products Ltd, Plymouth, PL3 5UA.

G.F. Dietary Supplies Ltd, 7 Queensbury Station Parade, Queensbury, Edgware, Middlesex, HA8 5NP.

Montedison Pharmaceuticals Ltd., Station Road, Barnet, Herts, EN5 1NU.

Procea Ltd., Alexandra Road, Dublin.

Welfare Foods (Stockport) Ltd., 63 London Road South, Poynton, Stockport, Cheshire, SK12 1LA.

The packaging of products which are gluten free is marked with this symbol by the manufacturer.

In some areas gluten free bread is made locally.

A recipe for a gluten free raising agent is given below:

Gluten free raising agent

Ingredients: 20 g baking soda
40 g cream of tartar
60 g cornflour

Method of preparation: Mix all ingredients and pass four times through a fine sieve. Store in an air-tight container.

The Coeliac Society, P.O. Box 181, London, NW2 2QY

This society produces lists of manufactured foods which are gluten free. Care must be taken to ensure that the most recently produced list is used because the recipes used for products are often changed. The Coeliac Society also publish other literature of interest to coeliacs and has local branches.

CARBOHYDRATE INTOLERANCE

Disaccharidase deficiency

This section deals with a particular aspect of the malabsorption syndrome, a prominent feature in this case being the presence in the intestine of unabsorbed carbohydrate. This condition is not infrequently seen in infancy when it causes diarrhoea with bulky or frothy acid stools and failure to thrive, and may prove fatal if untreated.

Normally, carbohydrate digestion proceeds as shown below, the simple sugars (monosaccharides) being finally absorbed into the body.

A common cause of carbohydrate intolerance is insufficient activity of one or more of the disaccharide-splitting enzymes or disaccharidases, maltase, isomaltase, sucrase and lactase, resulting in the presence in the bowel of the appropriate disaccharide in abnormally large amount. This enzyme deficiency may be due to temporary immaturity for a period following birth or may be secondary to disease of the bowel such as coeliac disease or gastroenteritis. Carbohydrate intolerance due to an inborn defect involving carbohydrate-digesting enzymes occurs, although more rarely. Failure to absorb monosaccharides has also been reported. Treatment consists of omitting the offending material from the diet.

Carbohydrate digestion

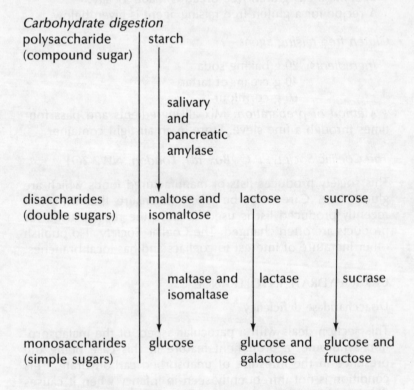

polysaccharide (compound sugar)	starch		
	salivary and pancreatic amylase		
disaccharides (double sugars)	maltose and isomaltose	lactose	sucrose
	maltase and isomaltase	lactase	sucrase
monosaccharides (simple sugars)	glucose	glucose and galactose	glucose and fructose

It should be noted that starch is the principal dietary source of maltose and isomaltose.

If improvement takes place on a lactose free (milk free) diet, as described in the section on galactosaemia, this diet may be continued until the child is sufficiently recovered for confirmatory tests to be done. The position may however be more complex, involving several enzymes; for instance infants who cannot digest lactose sometimes cannot digest sucrose either. It is possible to carry out investigations which will indicate the exact nature of the defect. If the child is too ill to undergo these a disaccharide free, starch free diet must be instituted without delay and the tests postponed until later. It is possible to give a carbohydrate free diet for a time if necessary. Certain milk substitutes and proprietary foods suitable for the treatment of carbohydrate intolerance are described below.

The diet must be adequate in respect of all essential food factors, including minerals and vitamins. Mineral or vitamin tablets often contain a carbohydrate filler and many preparations are administered in syrup form. Ketovite Tablets and Liquid (Paines and Byrne Ltd.) provide a complete vitamin supplement and are carbohydrate free.

Expansion of the diet

When the exact nature of the intolerance is known the child may be found to tolerate certain of the suspect carbohydrates and the diet may be extended. For success it is necessary to have the detailed supervision of a dietitian or other person with specialised knowledge of the composition of foods. Hardinge, Swarner and Crooks* have compiled a useful tabulation of carbohydrates found in a wide variety of foods, as also have Southgate, Paul, Dean and Christie†.

MILK SUBSTITUTES AND PROPRIETARY FOODS SUITABLE FOR THE TREATMENT OF MALABSORPTION

When malabsorption occurs in infancy the selection of a suitable formula can prove difficult. Some examples of specialised proprietary foods suitable for this purpose are described

* Hardinge, M.G., Swarner, J.B. and Crooks, H. (1965). *J. Amer. Diet. Ass.*, **46**, 3, 197
† Southgate, D.A.T., Paul, Alison A., Dean, Ann C. and Christie, A.A. (1978. *J. Hum. Nutr.*, **32**, 5, 335.

below. Certain of these foods contain medium chain triglycerides (MCT), which are described in Chapter 23. Some contain protein in hydrolysed form; this is an indication that the proteins have been either partly or completely split into their constituent amino acids, in which form they require the minimum of digestion and are therefore more readily absorbed into the body. The significance of the nature of the carbohydrate content has been discussed above. All are free from gluten.

The details given below are not exhaustive, and in each case further information should be obtained from the manufacturer.

Galactomin (Cow and Gate) is available in three forms. *Galactomin 17* and *Reduced Fat Galactomin 18* are devoid of sucrose and contain only traces of lactose. *Galactomin 19* is similar to Reduced Fat Galactomin 18 in composition, being a low fat food with only a trace of lactose; in this case the only other carbohydrate is fructose. Galactomin 19 is intended for use when failure to absorb the monosaccharides glucose and/or galactose is suspected.

Nutramigen (Mead Johnson) contains carbohydrate as starch and sucrose, and has a trace only of lactose. It should not be used when there is intolerance of both lactose and sucrose. The protein (casein) is in hydrolysed form.

Formula MCT (1) (Cow and Gate) contains fat in the form of MCT oil, is low in lactose and free from sucrose.

Portagen Powder (Mead Johnson) contains fat partly in the form of medium chain triglycerides and carbohydrate as sugar (sucrose) and corn syrup solids. It has a trace of lactose.

Pregestimil (Mead Johnson) is devoid of lactose or sucrose and contains protein principally as hydrolysed casein. Fat is 40 per cent MCT oil and 60 per cent corn oil.

Velactin (A. Wander Ltd.) and *ProSobee (Mead Johnson)* are milk substitutes based on the soya bean. Both are free from lactose. Neither contains added sucrose.

A synthetic feed requiring the minimum of digestion can be devised, based on a hydrolysed protein preparation such as 'Albumaid' Hydrolysate Complete, with Maxijul, MCT oil and Metabolic Mineral Mixture (all from Scientific Hospital Supplies Ltd.), and a complete vitamin supplement such as Ketovite Tablets and Liquid (Paines and Byrne Ltd.). A source of essential fatty acids, such as corn oil, should be included.

This is an example of an elemental diet as described in Chapter 23. In this case the components, carbohydrate, minerals, protein etc. are assembled when the mixture is required. Final composition is therefore more flexible than in the case of a prepacked complete feed such as Vivonex.

Vitamin and mineral supplements

In the use of specialised foods such as those listed above the manufacturer's literature should be studied carefully, as some require supplementation with minerals and vitamins. It should be noted also that many drugs and vitamin preparations are in syrup form, and that tablets often contain a carbohydrate filler. Ketovite Tablets and Liquid (Paines and Byrne Ltd.) provide a complete vitamin supplement and are carbohydrate free. Supplementary Vitamin Tablets for infants (Cow and Gate) contain certain vitamins and trace elements, are lactose free but contain sucrose.

GALACTOSAEMIA

Galactosaemia is an inherited disorder of galactose metabolism. In normal persons the simple sugar galactose is converted to glucose in the body as a result of a series of chemical reactions, each of which requires the presence of a specific enzyme. In galactosaemia the enzyme which promotes the second stage of this conversion is lacking. This gives rise to accumulation in the tissues of galactose and an intermediate conversion product, galactose-1-phosphate, causing damage to the brain, liver and kidneys, and to the lens of the eye, resulting in cataract. In seriously affected cases vomiting, refusal of food, loss of weight and jaundice are apparent during the first few days or weeks of life, the condition usually proving fatal if treatment is delayed.

Diet

The only dietary source of galactose is milk sugar or lactose, which yields glucose and galactose on digestion. Thus in galactosaemia milk and milk products must be excluded from the diet. A suitable milk substitute could be selected from the foods already listed in this chapter for the treatment of malabsorption. It should be noted, however, that in this case it is only necessary to consider a minimal lactose content. A comprehensive vitamin supplement may be required, depending upon the composition of the food selected.

Lactose in pharmaceutical preparations

Lactose is frequently used as a filler in the preparation of tablets (including ascorbic acid tablets), lozenges and pastilles. For this reason such preparations are not prescribed for patients with galactosaemia unless their detailed composition is known.

Supplementary Vitamin Tablets for infants (Cow and Gate) may be given in conjunction with this diet, as also may Ketovite Tablets and Liquid (Paines and Byrne Ltd.). In the case of the former product vitamins A and D may be required in addition, and can be conveniently supplied from cod liver oil or other fish liver oil. Ketovite Tablets and Liquid are complementary and do not duplicate one another.

Mixed feeding

Following the introduction of mixed feeding, care should be taken to exclude any foods likely to contain traces of milk.

Some examples of foods to avoid, or details sought as to their composition

Milk, cheese, ice cream, butter and margarine.
Milk loaf, and any bought breads, biscuits, cakes and pastries unless known to be free from milk.
Prepared cake and pudding mixes. Proprietary infant foods.
Breakfast cereals.
Canned or packet soups and sauces. Sandwich spreads.
Confectionery. Lemon curd.

Foods permitted

Most standard plain or pan loaves—confirmation should be sought from baker.

Unmixed starchy foods such as cornflour, rice, semolina, oatmeal, sago and tapioca.

Vegetable oils and cooking fats, lard, dripping and Outline Low Fat Spread (Van den Berghs).

Fresh meat, fish and eggs.

Fresh, frozen or dried vegetables, or vegetables canned in brine.

Fresh, frozen, canned or dried fruit.

Fruit juices and fruit syrups.

Jam, marmalade, honey and syrup.

Tea, coffee made from coffee grounds, minerals.

Where proprietary foods are concerned lactose free varieties are frequently available. Most manufacturers will supply information on request.

Sucrose intolerance

All dietary sources of sucrose (sugar) are excluded.

Fructose intolerance

Sucrose is digested to fructose and glucose and so must be excluded from the diet. Fructose occurs naturally in fruit, therefore fruit must also be excluded.

PHENYLKETONURIA

Phenylketonuria is a rare disease resulting from inability to metabolise normally the amino acid phenylalanine.

We have already seen (Chapter 4) that proteins are composed of amino acid units, and that the amino acids from dietary proteins provide the materials from which are constructed the proteins of the body tissues and fluids, any not required for structural purposes being broken down to yield energy. During these metabolic processes any phenylalanine not required as such by the tissues is converted to another amino acid, tyrosine. In persons with phenylketonuria this transformation does not take place owing to lack of a specific enzyme, with the result that phenylalanine, and

certain abnormal breakdown products known as phenylke-
tones, accumulate in the body fluids and are excreted in the
urine. The presence of these constituents in the body fluids
results in nervous system abnormalities including progressive
brain damage. In some cases skin lesions also occur. Infants
with phenylketonuria have normal blood phenylalanine levels
at birth. Raised levels follow the introduction of milk feeds.
Accumulation of harmful metabolites may become apparent
any time between the first and the sixth weeks. Early diagnosis
is of the utmost importance, as there is evidence that initiation
of treatment before brain damage occurs can prevent the
development of mental deficiency.

Phenylalanine is necessary for the structure of body
proteins, and as it cannot be manufactured in the body it must
be supplied in the diet. A normal diet, however, supplies
amino acids, including phenylalanine, in excess of the body's
requirements. Since the object of treatment of phenylketonuria is to prevent accumulation in the body of phenylalanine
and its abnormal derivatives, treatment consists in providing
a diet low in phenylalanine, containing only the amount of
this amino acid which can be utilised by the tissues. A lack of
tyrosine need not necessarily occur as this amino acid is also
obtained from the diet.

Diet

In the construction of a low phenylalanine diet the greater
part of the protein must be obtained from a synthetic
preparation of low phenylalanine content. Phenylalanine requirements are met by adding measured amounts of protein-
containing foods until the individuals tolerance of this amino
acid has been reached. Some proprietary foods which may be
used as the basis of the diet are Minafen (Cow and Gate Ltd),
Lofenalac (Mead Johnson), Cymogran and Aminogran (Allen
and Hanburys Ltd), and Albumaid XP (Scientific Hospital·
Supplies Ltd.). In the case of infants the selected proprietary
food is used as the basis of a feeding mixture, the necessary
phenylalanine being added in the form of measured amounts
of milk. Supplements of carbohydrate, fat, minerals and vitamins will depend upon the composition of the food selected.
Ketovite Tablets and Liquid (Paines and Byrne Ltd), taken

together, provide complete supplementation for synthetic diets. A metabolic mineral mixture is available from Scientific Hospital Supplies Ltd, and Allen and Hanburys Ltd. Fat is conveniently supplied by Prosparol and carbohydrate as Caloreen or Maxijul; these are described in Chapter 21.

In the majority of cases a phenylalanine allowance of 50 mg per kg body weight may be given to begin with, subsequent adjustments being based on blood phenylalanine estimations. In some cases requirement may be considerably in excess of this figure, and since dietary deficiency of phenylalanine also gives rise to mental retardation caution is required. Blood should be carefully monitored, especially during the first few weeks, the aim being to maintain a level of between 125 and 375 μmol per l.

For older children the milk is replaced by a small allowance of ordinary food, which must be measured. Some suitable milk replacements are listed below. As the allowance of ordinary food is usually very small, in many cases equivalent to around 200 mg phenylalanine daily, the bulk of the diet consists of low protein pasta, flour, bread and biscuits. These foods are used also in low protein diets for kidney failure and are listed on page 257. Prosparol can be mixed with water and Caloreen to give a milk substitute which can be added to tea, poured over breakfast cereal, and made into a pudding with cornflour or custard powder, which are unrestricted.

As the child gets older the brain becomes less susceptible to damage by the abnormal metabolites and it is usual to permit some relaxation of the diet. Opinions differ as to the age at which this should take place. At around seven or eight years has been advocated. The diet will then contain a much greater allowance of natural food, principally in the form of cereals and vegetables. Blood phenylalanine levels are still subject to control, although at a higher level than formerly, and it may be necessary to include a small supplement of the special protein food.

Classification of foods for low phenylalanine diets

The classification given below aims at combining adequate control of phenylalanine intake with a minimum of restrictions. The average helpings specified for the second group of foods should be strictly adhered to, as some vegetables and fruits included in this group contribute very significantly to the phenylalanine intake.

These items may be taken in unrestricted amounts:

sugar	vegetable cooking fats and
clear boiled sweets	oils
syrup	tea and coffee
honey	minerals and squashes
jam and marmalade	flavouring essences
butter and margarine	spices and condiments
lard	cornflour and custard powder
	sago, arrowroot and tapioca

vegetable cooking water, for example cabbage, carrot or celery cooking water. Low protein flour, bread and other items listed on p. 257.

These may be taken in unweighed average helpings:

green vegetables	tomatoes and tomato juice
root vegetables except potatoes	fruit juices
fruit except dried fruit	

Some examples of foods which must be measured. They can be exchanged for each other in the portions stated. Each portion supplies approximately 50 mg phenylalanine:

ordinary bread	15 g	potato boiled	80 g
biscuits	15 g	potato chips	30 g
cornflakes	15 g	potato crisps, plain	20 g
Rice Krispies	15 g	peas or broad beans,	
oatmeal	10 g	fresh boiled	30 g
ice cream	20 g	rice boiled in water	40 g
milk	30 ml		
double cream	60 ml		
whipping cream	40 ml		

Other disorders of amino acid metabolism occur but very infrequently. In some conditions, it may be necessary to control the intake of more than one amino acid, for example, in maple syrup urine disease the intakes of valine, leucine and isoleucine are all restricted. These three amino acids are also essential amino acids and cannot be completely excluded from the diet.

Conclusion

Having a child on a special diet imposes many restrictions and strains on the family. For example, treats like an ice cream at the seaside, or a visit to a friend's home for tea are often impossible. It is important that everybody involved in that child's care understands the diet. This includes grandparents, child minders, nurses and health visitors.

QUESTIONS

1. Explain the dietary restrictions necessary in gluten-sensitive enteropathy?
2. Suggest a day's menu for a 3 year old with gluten sensitive enteropathy who will not eat gluten free bread.
3. One of the symptoms of carbohydrate intolerance is diarrhoea. How is this caused?
4. What are the principles of dietary treatment of children with disorders of amino acid metabolism?

Further reading

Cameron Margaret, Hofvander Yngve 1976 Manual on feeding infants and young children, 2nd edn. FAO/WHO/UNICEF Protein Advisory Group of the United Nations System, New York, p 184

Dept. of Health and Social Security 1979 Report on Health and Social Subjects 15. Recommended daily amounts of food energy and nutrients for groups of people in the United Kingdom. H.M.S.O., London

Dept. of Health and Social Security 1979 Prevention and health. Eating for Health. H.M.S.O., London.

Mayer Jean, Dwyer Johanna T 1979 Food and nutrition policy in a changing world, 1st edn. Oxford University Press, New York.

Francis Dorothy E M 1974 Diets for sick children, 3rd edn. Blackwell, Oxford and Edinburgh,

Good housekeeping basic cookery 1976 Ebury Press, London

Hobbs Betty C, Gilbert R J 1978 Food poisoning and food hygiene, 4th edn. Arnold, London, p 366

McKeith R, Wood C 1977 Infant feeding and feeding difficulties, 5th edn. Churchill Livingstone, London, p 330

Ministry of Agriculture, Fisheries and Food 1976 Manual of Nutrition, 8th edn. H.M.S.O., London,

Mottram R F 1979 Human nutrition, 3rd edn. Arnold, London, p 179

Patten Marguerite 1976 Learning to cook, 2nd edn. Pan Books, London, p 220

Paul A A, Southgate D A T 1978 The composition of foods, 4th edn. MRC Special Report No. 297. H.M.S.O., London, p 418

Which? 1978 Way to slim. Consumers' Association, London.

Journals

Nutrition and Food Science, Bi-monthly. Forbes, London

Journal of Human Nutrition, Bi-monthly. John Libbey, London

Information Bulletins, published January, May, September: The British Nutrition Foundation, 15 Belgrave Square, London SW1X 8PS

Appendices

APPENDIX 1

UNITS OF MEASUREMENT

Weight

1000 micrograms (μg)	= 1 milligram (mg)
1000 milligrams	= 1 gram (g)
1000 grams	= 1 kilogram (kg)

28.35 grams (30 approx)	= 1 ounce
1 kilogram	= 2.205 pounds (2.2 approx)

Volume

1000 millilitres (ml)	= 1 litre (l)

28.4 millilitres (30 approx)	= 1 fluid ounce (fl oz)
568 millilitres (550 approx)	= 1 pint (p)
1 litre	= 1.76 pints (1¾ approx)

1 teacup = 150 ml = 5 fluid ounces ⎫
⎬ Approximately
1 glass = 225 ml = 8 fluid ounces ⎭

Energy
4.184 joules (4.2 approx.) = 1 calorie

APPENDIX 2

RECOMMENDED DAILY AMOUNTS OF FOOD ENERGY AND SOME NUTRIENTS FOR POPULATION GROUPS IN THE UNITED KINGDOM

Age range(a) years	Occupational category	Energy MJ	Energy Kcal	Protein g	Thiamin mg	Riboflavin mg
Boys						
under 1		(b)	(b)	(b)	0.3	0.4
1		5.0	1200	30	0.5	0.6
2		5.75	1400	35	0.6	0.7
3–4		6.5	1560	39	0.6	0.8
5–6		7.25	1740	43	0.7	0.9
7–8		8.25	1980	49	0.8	1.0
9–11		9.5	2280	57	0.9	1.2
12–14		11.0	2640	66	1.1	1.4
15–17		12.0	2880	72	1.2	1.7
Girls						
under 1		(b)	(b)	(b)	0.3	0.4
1		4.5	1100	27	0.4	0.6
2		5.5	1300	32	0.5	0.7
3–4		6.25	1500	37	0.6	0.8
5–6		7.0	1680	42	0.7	0.9
7–8		8.0	1900	47	0.8	1.0
9–11		8.5	2050	51	0.8	1.2
12–14		9.0	2150	53	0.9	1.4
15–17		9.0	2150	53	0.9	1.7
Men						
18–34	Sedentary	10.5	2510	63	1.0	1.6
	Moderately active	12.0	2900	72	1.2	1.6
	Very active	14.0	3350	84	1.3	1.6
35–64	Sedentary	10.0	2400	60	1.0	1.6
	Moderately active	11.5	2750	69	1.1	1.6
	Very active	14.0	3350	84	1.3	1.6
65–74	Assuming a	10.0	2400	60	1.0	1.6
75+	sedentary life	9.0	2150	54	0.9	1.6
Women						
18–54	Most occupations	9.0	2150	54	0.9	1.3
	Very active	10.5	2500	62	1.0	1.3
55–74	Assuming a	8.0	1900	47	0.8	1.3
75+	sedentary life	7.0	1680	42	0.7	1.3
Pregnancy		10.0	2400	60	1.0	1.6
Lactation		11.5	2750	69	1.1	1.8

Notes to Table

a Since the recommendations are average amounts, the figures for each age range represent the amounts recommended at the middle of the range. Within each age range, younger children will need less, and older children more, than the amount recommended.
b Figures for protein and energy for children under 1 year; see original Report.
c No information is available about requirements for children for folate. Graded amounts are recommended between the figure shown for infants under 1 year, which is based upon the average folate content of mature human milk, and the 300 μg daily which is suggested for adults.

The Committee on Medical Aspects of Food Policy of the Department of Health and Social Services: Report on Health and Social Subjects 15, 1979. Reproduced by permission of the Controller of Her Majesty's Stationery Office. The original Report should be consulted for background information relating to the figures given here.

Nicotinic acid equivalents mg	Total folate(c) µg	Ascorbic acid mg	Vitamin A retinol equivalents µg	Vitamin D (d) cholecalciferol µg	Calcium mg	Iron mg
5	50	20	450	7.5	600	6
7	100	20	300	10	600	7
8	100	20	300	10	600	7
9	100	20	300	10	600	8
10	200	20	300	(d)	600	10
11	200	20	400	(d)	600	10
14	200	25	575	(d)	700	12
16	300	25	725	(d)	700	12
19	300	30	750	(d)	600	12
5	50	20	450	7.5	600	6
7	100	20	300	10	600	7
8	100	20	300	10	600	7
9	100	20	300	10	600	8
10	200	20	300	(d)	600	10
11	200	20	400	(d)	600	10
14	300	25	575	(d)	700	12(f)
16	300	25	725	(d)	700	12(f)
19	300	30	750	(d)	600	12(f)
18	300	30	750	(d)	500	10
18	300	30	750	(d)	500	10
18	300	30	750	(d)	500	10
18	300	30	750	(d)	500	10
18	300	30	750	(d)	500	10
18	300	30	750	(d)	500	10
18	300	30	750	(d)	500	10
18	300	30	750	(d)	500	10
15	300	30	750	(d)	500	12(f)
15	300	30	750		500	12(f)
15	300	30	750	(d)	500	10
15	300	30	750	(d)	500	10
18	500	60	750	10	1200(e)	13
21	400	60	1200	10	1200	15

d No dietary sources may be necessary for children and adults who are sufficiently exposed to sunlight, but during the winter children and adolescents should receive 10 µg (400 i.u.) daily by supplementation. Adults with inadequate exposure to sunlight, for example those who are housebound, may also need a supplement of 10 µg daily.

e For the third trimester only.

f This intake may not be sufficient for 10% of girls and women with large menstrual losses.

APPENDIX 3
DIETARY GUIDELINES FOR THE UK

DHSS (Department of Health and Social Security) 1978; revised 1979. Eating for health. HMSO, London. Reproduced by permission of the Controller of Her Majesty's Stationery Office.

1. If babies can be breast-fed even for a few days and preferably, for a few weeks or a few months, this gives them the best possible start in life.
2. As soon as solid foods are started dietary habits towards foods other than milk are formed. In particular, sweet foods may help a child to develop a 'sweet tooth', and perhaps eventually to lose his teeth due to dental caries; therefore, the use of sugar and confectionery should be limited.
3. During times of rapid growth—infancy and the pre-school years—sufficient vitamin D is important. Supplements may be needed during the winter, especially in towns. They may also be needed during puberty, pregnancy and when breast-feeding; the house-bound may also require them.
4. To ensure health the diet must provide enough energy, enough protein and enough of the minerals and vitamins. If the diet comprises a mixture of many different foods and includes cereal foods, protein foods, some fat (to ensure essential fatty acids), fruit and vegetables so that energy needs are met, then enough of all other essential nutrients will be provided.
5. Obesity can mean ill-health or premature death. To avoid these, food intake should not be greater than is necessary for energy expenditure. A practical way of ensuring this is not to become overweight for one's height.
6. People need to watch the amount of fats and sweet foods they eat. Many people need to cut down their intake of:
    visible fats in the form of cream, butter, margarine, fat on meat, fried foods;
    invisible fats in cakes, biscuits, puddings, pastry, ice cream;
    sugar in sweets, chocolate, puddings, soft drinks, tea, coffee and other beverages.
7. The reduction in energy intake which results from eating less fat and less sugar can be made up by eating more bread, and more fresh fruit and vegetables including potatoes. All these foods are less fattening, weight for weight, than the fatty sweet foods listed in 6.
8. It would do no harm for most people to eat a little less protein.
9. To eat less salt might be beneficial.
10. Alcohol is not a necessary food, and sweets, soft drinks, preserves and other confectionery are also unnecessary. These should be thought of as party foods.

APPENDIX 4

AVERAGE WEIGHTS FOR MEN AND WOMEN
ACCORDING TO HEIGHT AND AGE

Height (in shoes)[a] cm	Weight in kilograms (in indoor clothing)[b]					
	Ages 20 to 24	Ages 25 to 29	Ages 30 to 39	Ages 40 to 49	Ages 50 to 59	Ages 60 to 69
Men—						
158	58.1	60.8	62.1	63.5	64.4	63.0
160	59.9	62.6	64.0	65.3	65.8	64.4
163	61.7	64.0	65.8	67.1	67.6	66.2
165	63.0	65.3	67.6	68.9	69.4	68.0
168	64.4	67.1	69.4	70.8	71.2	69.9
170	65.8	68.5	71.2	73.0	73.5	72.1
173	67.6	70.3	73.0	74.8	75.3	73.9
175	69.4	72.1	74.8	76.7	77.1	76.2
178	71.2	73.9	77.1	78.9	79.4	78.5
180	73.0	75.7	78.9	80.7	81.6	80.7
183	75.3	78.0	81.2	83.0	83.9	83.0
185	77.1	80.3	83.0	84.8	85.7	85.3
188	78.9	82.6	85.3	87.1	88.0	87.5
191	80.7	84.4	87.5	89.4	90.3	89.8
193	82.1	86.2	90.3	92.1	93.0	92.5
Women—						
147	46.3	48.5	52.2	55.3	56.7	57.6
150	47.6	49.9	53.1	56.2	57.6	58.5
152	49.0	51.3	54.4	57.6	59.0	59.4
155	50.8	52.6	55.8	59.0	60.3	60.8
158	52.2	54.0	57.2	60.3	61.7	62.1
160	53.5	55.3	58.5	61.7	63.5	64.0
163	54.9	56.7	59.9	63.5	65.3	65.8
165	56.7	58.5	61.2	64.9	67.1	67.6
168	58.5	60.3	63.0	66.7	68.9	69.4
170	59.9	61.7	64.4	68.5	70.8	71.2
173	61.7	63.5	66.2	70.3	72.6	73.0
175	63.5	65.3	68.0	72.1	74.4	74.8
178	65.3	67.1	69.9	74.4	76.7	*
180	67.6	69.4	72.1	76.7	78.9	*
183	69.9	71.7	74.4	78.9	81.6	*

[a] 2.5-cm heels for men and 5-cm heels for women.
[b] 3.2 to 4.1 kg allowed for men, 1.8 to 2.7 kg for women.
* Average weights not determined because of insufficient data.
Source: Metric conversion of the figures from the Metropolitan Life Insurance Company (1960).

Appendix 4 — continued

DESIRABLE WEIGHTS FOR MEN AND WOMEN ACCORDING TO HEIGHT AND FRAME (AGES 25 AND OVER)

Height (in shoes)[a] cm	Weight in kilograms (in indoor clothing)[b]		
	Small frame	Medium frame	Large frame
Men—			
157	50.8 to 54.4	53.5 to 58.5	57.1 to 64.0
160	52.2 to 55.8	54.9 to 60.3	58.5 to 65.3
163	53.5 to 57.2	56.2 to 61.7	59.9 to 67.1
165	54.9 to 58.5	57.6 to 63.0	61.2 to 68.9
168	56.2 to 60.3	59.0 to 64.9	62.6 to 70.8
170	58.1 to 62.1	60.8 to 66.7	64.4 to 73.0
173	59.9 to 64.0	62.6 to 68.9	66.7 to 75.3
175	61.7 to 65.8	64.4 to 70.8	68.5 to 77.1
178	63.5 to 68.0	66.2 to 72.6	70.3 to 78.9
180	65.3 to 69.9	68.0 to 74.8	72.1 to 81.2
183	67.1 to 71.7	69.9 to 77.1	74.4 to 83.5
185	68.9 to 73.5	71.7 to 79.4	76.2 to 85.7
188	70.8 to 75.8	73.5 to 81.6	78.5 to 88.0
191	72.6 to 77.6	75.7 to 83.9	80.7 to 90.3
193	74.4 to 79.4	78.0 to 86.2	82.6 to 92.5
Women—			
147	41.7 to 44.5	43.5 to 48.5	47.2 to 54.0
150	42.6 to 45.8	44.5 to 49.9	48.1 to 55.3
152	43.5 to 47.2	45.8 to 51.3	49.4 to 56.7
155	44.9 to 48.5	47.2 to 52.6	50.8 to 58.1
157	46.3 to 49.9	48.5 to 54.0	52.2 to 59.4
160	47.6 to 51.3	49.9 to 55.3	53.5 to 60.8
163	49.0 to 52.6	51.3 to 57.2	54.9 to 62.6
165	50.3 to 54.0	52.6 to 59.0	56.7 to 64.4
168	51.7 to 55.8	54.4 to 61.2	58.5 to 66.2
170	53.5 to 57.6	56.2 to 63.0	60.3 to 68.0
173	55.3 to 59.4	58.1 to 64.9	62.1 to 69.9
175	57.2 to 61.2	59.9 to 66.7	64.0 to 71.7
178	59.0 to 63.5	61.7 to 68.5	65.8 to 73.9
180	60.8 to 65.3	63.5 to 70.3	67.6 to 76.2
183	62.6 to 67.1	65.3 to 72.1	69.4 to 78.9

[a] 2.5-cm heels for men and 5-cm heels for women.
[b] 3.2 to 4.1 kg allowed for men, 1.8 to 2.7 kg for women.
Note: A metric conversion from figures prepared by the Metropolitan Life Insurance Company (1960), derived primarily from data of the Build and Blood Pressure Study, 1959.

Appendix 4 — continued

HEIGHTS AND WEIGHT OF BRITISH CHILDREN, 1965[a]

	Boys		Girls	
Age	Height (supine Length up to 2 years)	Weight	Height (supine length up to 2 years)	Weight
yr	cm	kg	cm	kg
0.25	60.7	5.93	59.0	5.56
0.50	68.2	7.90	65.5	7.39
0.75	72.7	9.20	70.2	8.72
1.00	76.3	10.2	74.2	9.7
1.25	79.4	11.0	77.6	10.4
1.50	82.1	11.6	80.5	11.1
1.75	84.6	12.2	83.2	11.7
2.00	86.9	12.7	85.6	12.2
2.5	90.2	13.7	88.9	13.3
3.0	94.2	14.7	93.0	14.3
4.0	101.6	16.6	100.4	16.3
5.0	108.3	18.5	107.2	18.3
6.0	114.6	20.5	113.4	20.4
7.0	120.5	22.6	119.3	22.6
8.0	126.2	25.0	125.0	25.1
9.0	131.6	27.5	130.6	27.7
10.0	136.8	30.3	136.4	31.1
11.0	141.9	33.6	142.7	35.2
12.0	147.3	37.7	149.3	40.5
13.0	153.4	42.6	155.5	45.8
14.0	160.7	48.8	159.6	51.0
15.0	167.3	54.7	161.7	54.4
16.0	172.2	59.6	162.2	55.8
17.0	174.3	61.9	..	56.4
18.0	174.7	63.0	..	56.6
19.0	..	63.3	..	56.7

With acknowledgement of the Authors, Editor and Publisher of *Standards from birth to maturity for height, weight, height velocity and weight velocity: British children*, 1965, by J. M. Tanner, R. H. Whitehouse and M. Takaishi (1966). *Arch. Dis. Chldh.*, **41**, 454.
[a] Principally London.

APPENDIX 5

COMPOSITION OF FOODS per 100 GRAMS

These figures are crown copyright material, taken from *The Composition of Foods* by A. A. Paul and D. A. T. Southgate, fourth, revised and extended edition of MRC Special Report No 297, and reproduced by permission of the Controller of Her Majesty's Stationery Office.

This Report should be consulted for further information relating to the composition of foods, to the figures quoted here, and for the recipes used in the preparation of the cooked dishes for which figures have been given. The following symbols have been employed:

O   Signifies that virtually none of the constituent is known to be present

Tr   Indicates that a trace is known to be present

( )   Figures in parentheses are estimates taken from related foods, or more rarely, tentative values based on a limited number of published sources.

—   A dash shows that no information is available.

Food	Energy value kcal	Energy value kJ	Protein g	Fat g	Carbo-hydrate g	Sodium mg	Potassium mg	Calcium mg	Iron mg	Dietary fibre g
Cereals and cereal products										
Grains, flours and starches										
Bran wheat	206	872	14.1	5.5	26.8	28	1160	110	12.9	44
Cornflour	354	1508	0.6	0.7	92.0	52	61	15	1.4	—
Custard powder	354	1508	0.6	0.7	92.0	320	61	15	1.4	—
Flour wholemeal (100%)	318	1351	13.2	2.0	65.8	3	360	35	4.0	9.6
brown (85%)	327	1392	12.8	2.0	68.8	4	280	150	3.6	7.5
white (72%) breadmaking	337	1433	11.3	1.2	74.8	3	130	140	2.2	3.0
household, plain	350	1493	9.8	1.2	80.1	2	140	150	2.4	3.4

Cereals and cereal products (continued)

Macaroni boiled in water, unsalted	117	499	4.3	0.6	25.2	8	67	8	0.5	—
Oatmeal Porridge	44	188	1.4	0.9	8.2	580	42	6	0.5	0.8
Rice polished, raw	361	1536	6.5	1.0	86.8	6	110	4	0.5	2.4
boiled in water, unsalted	123	522	2.2	0.3	29.6	2	38	1	0.2	0.8
Spaghetti canned in tomato sauce	59	250	1.7	0.7	12.2	500	130	21	0.4	—
Bread										
Bread wholemeal	216	918	8.8	2.7	41.8	540	220	23	2.5	8.5
brown	223	948	8.9	2.2	44.7	550	210	100	2.5	5.1
Hovis	228	968	9.7	2.2	45.1	580	210	150	4.5	4.6
white	233	991	7.8	1.7	49.7	540	100	100	1.7	2.7
Chapatis made with fat	336	1415	8.1	12.8	50.2	130	160	66	2.3	3.7
made without fat	202	860	7.3	1.0	43.7	120	150	60	2.1	(3.4)
Breakfast cereals										
All-bran (Kellogg's)	273	1156	15.1	5.7	43.0	1670	1070	74	12.0	26.7
Cornflakes (Kellogg's)	368	1567	8.6	1.6	85.1	1160	99	3	0.6	1.38
Ready Brek (Lyons)	390	1651	12.4	8.7	69.9	23	390	64	4.9	7.6
Rice Krispies (Kellogg's)	372	1584	5.9	2.0	88.1	1110	160	7	0.7	4.5
Shredded Wheat (Nabisco)	324	1378	10.6	3.0	67.9	8	330	38	4.2	12.3
Weetabix (Weetabix)	340	1444	11.4	3.4	70.3	360	420	33	7.6	12.7

| Food | Energy value | | Protein | Fat | Carbo-hydrate | mg | | | | Dietary fibre |
	kcal	kJ	g	g	g	Sodium	Potassium	Calcium	Iron	g
Biscuits										
Cream crackers	440	1857	9.5	16.3	68.3	610	120	110	1.7	(3.0)
Digestive plain	471	1981	9.8	20.5	66.0	440	160	110	2.0	(5.5)
chocolate	493	2071	6.8	24.1	66.5	450	210	84	2.1	3.5
Matzo	384	1634	10.5	1.9	86.6	17	150	32	1.5	3.9
Semi-sweet	457	1925	6.7	16.6	74.8	410	140	120	2.1	2.3
Cakes										
Fancy iced cakes	407	1717	3.8	14.9	68.8	250	170	44	1.4	2.4
Fruit cake rich	332	1403	3.7	11.0	58.3	170	430	75	1.8	3.5
Madeira cake	393	1652	5.4	16.9	58.4	380	120	42	1.1	1.4
Buns and pastries										
Doughnuts	349	1467	6.0	15.8	48.8	60	110	70	1.9	—
Pastry, shortcrust cooked	527	2202	6.9	32.2	55.8	480	99	110	1.8	2.4
Scones	371	1562	7.5	14.6	55.9	800	140	620	1.5	2.1
Puddings										
Apple crumble	208	878	1.8	6.9	37.0	68	100	28	0.6	2.5
Cheesecake	421	1747	4.2	34.9	24.0	260	120	67	0.7	0.9
Custard egg	118	497	5.8	6.0	11.0	78	170	130	0.5	—
made with powder	118	496	3.8	4.4	16.8	76	170	140	0.1	—
Fruit pie individual, with pastry top and bottom	369	1554	4.3	15.5	56.7	210	120	51	1.2	2.6
Ice cream dairy	167	704	3.7	6.6	24.8	80	180	140	0.2	—
non-dairy	165	691	3.3	8.2	20.7	70	150	120	0.3	—
Jelly packet, cubes	259	1104	6.1	0	62.5	25	25	32	1.7	—
made with water	59	251	1.4	0	14.2	6	6	7	0.4	—
Sponge pudding steamed	344	1443	5.9	16.4	46.0	310	88	210	1.2	1.2
Trifle	160	674	3.5	6.1	24.3	50	150	82	0.7	—

Milk and milk products

Milk, cows'

						50 (35–90)	150 (110–170)	120 (110–130)	0.05 (0.03–0.06)
fresh, whole	65	272	3.3	3.8	4.7	50	150	120	0.05
fresh, skimmed	33	142	3.4	0.1	5.0	52	150	130	0.05
condensed, whole, sweetened	332	1362	8.3	9.0	55.5	130	390	280	0.20
evaporated, whole, unsweetened	158	660	8.6	9.0	11.3	180	390	280	0.20
dried, whole	490	2051	26.3	26.3	39.4	440	1270	1020	0.40
Milk, human mature	69	289	1.3	4.1	7.2	14	58	34	0.07
Butter salted	740	3041	0.4	82.0	Tr	870	15	15	0.16

Cream

double	447	1841	1.5	48.2	2.0	27	79	50	0.20
whipping	332	1367	1.9	35.0	2.5	34	100	63	0.25

Cheese

Cheddar type (hard cheese)	406	1682	26.0	33.5	Tr	610	120	800	0.40
Cottage cheese	96	402	13.6	4.0	1.4	450	54	60	0.10
Cream cheese	439	1807	3.1	47.4	Tr	300	160	98	0.12
Processed cheese	311	1291	21.5	25.0	Tr	1360	82	700	0.50

Yogurt low fat

natural	52	216	5.0	1.0	6.2	76	240	180	0.09
flavoured	81	342	5.0	0.9	14.0	64	220	170	0.16
fruit	95	405	4.8	1.0	17.9	64	220	160	0.24

| Food | Energy value | | Protein | Fat | Carbo-hydrate | mg | | | | Dietary fibre |
	kcal	kJ	g	g	g	Sodium	Potassium	Calcium	Iron	g
Eggs										
Eggs whole, raw	147	612	12.3	10.9	Tr	140	140	52	2.0	
white, raw	36	153	9.0	Tr	Tr	190	150	5	0.1	
yolk, raw	339	1402	16.1	30.5	Tr	50	120	130	6.1	
fried	232	961	14.1	19.5	Tr	220	180	64	2.5	
Egg and cheese dishes										
Cauliflower cheese	113	471	5.7	8.0	4.9	250	250	160	0.4	
Macaroni cheese	174	726	7.4	9.7	15.1	280	120	180	0.4	
Quiche Lorraine	391	1627	14.7	28.1	21.1	610	190	260	1.3	
Scotch egg	279	1159	11.6	20.9	11.8	480	150	56	1.7	
Fats and oils										
Butter salted	740	3041	0.4	82.0	Tr	870	15	15	0.2	
Compound cooking fat	894	3674	Tr	99.3	0	Tr	Tr	Tr	Tr	
Lard	891	3663	Tr	99.0	0	2	1	1	0.1	
Low fat spread	366	1506	0	40.7	0	690	Tr	TR	Tr	
Margarine all kinds										
hard, soft and polyunsaturated	730	3000	0.1	81.0	0.1	800	5	4	0.3	
Vegetable oils	899	3696	Tr	99.9	0	Tr	Tr	Tr	Tr	

Meat and meat products

| Food | Energy value | | Protein | Fat | Carbo-hydrate | mg | | | | Dietary fibre |
	kcal	kJ	g	g	g	Sodium	Potassium	Calcium	Iron	g
Bacon rashers, grilled										
back, lean and fat	405	1681	25.3	33.8	0	2020	290	12	1.5	
streaky, lean and fat	422	1749	24.5	36.0	0	1990	290	12	1.5	

Beef									
brisket boiled, lean and fat, salt added	326	1354	27.6	23.9	0	73	200	12	2.8
mince stewed	229	955	23.1	15.2	0	320	290	18	3.1
rump steak fried, lean and fat	246	1026	28.6	14.6	0	54	360	7	3.2
silverside salted, boiled, lean only	173	730	32.3	4.9	0	1000	230	10	3.2
sirloin roast, lean and fat	284	1182	23.6	21.1	0	54	300	10	1.9
stewing steak, raw, lean and fat	176	736	20.2	10.6	0	72	320	8	2.1
Lamb									
cutlets, grilled, (weighed with bone)	244	1013	15.2	20.4	0	47	210	(6)	1.3
leg roast, lean and fat	266	1106	26.1	17.9	0	65	310	8	2.5
Pork									
chops, loin grilled (weighed with bone)	258	1073	22.2	18.8	0	66	300	(9)	0.9
leg roast, lean and fat	286	1190	26.9	19.8	0	79	350	10	1.3
Veal									
Fillet roast	230	963	31.6	11.5	0	97	430	14	1.6
Poultry									
Chicken roast									
light meat	142	599	26.5	4.0	0	71	330	9	0.5
dark meat	155	648	23.1	6.9	0	91	290	9	1.0
Duck roast, meat only weighed	189	789	25.3	9.7	0	96	270	13	2.7
Offal									
Kidney, lamb fried	155	651	24.6	6.3	0	270	340	13	12.0
Liver, calf, fried	254	1063	26.9	13.2	7.3	170	410	15	7.5
Tongue, ox pickled, raw	220	914	15.7	17.5	0	1210	300	7	4.9
boiled	293	1216	19.5	23.9	0	1000	150	31	3.0

Food	Energy value kcal	Energy value kJ	Protein g	Fat g	Carbohydrate g	Sodium mg	Potassium mg	Calcium mg	Iron mg	Dietary fibre g
Meat products and dishes										
Beef, corned, canned	217	905	26.9	12.1	0	950	140	14	2.9	
Ham, canned	120	502	18.4	5.1	0	1250	280	9	1.2	
Ham and pork chopped, canned	270	1118	14.4	23.6	0	1090	230	14	1.2	
Stewed steak with gravy, canned	176	730	14.8	12.5	1.0	380	240	14	2.1	
Salami	491	2031	19.3	45.2	1.9	1850	160	10	1.0	
Sausages pork, fried	317	1317	13.8	24.5	11.0	1050	200	55	1.5	
Beefburgers frozen, fried	264	1099	20.4	17.3	7.0	880	340	33	3.1	
Sausage roll flaky pastry	479	1991	7.2	36.2	33.1	550	110	70	1.3	
Beef stew	119	498	9.6	7.5	3.6	400	200	19	1.2	
Hot pot	114	480	9.3	4.2	10.4	670	430	22	1.2	
Shepherd's pie	119	497	7.6	6.1	8.9	450	240	15	1.1	
Fish and fish products										
Cod, baked, fillet, unsalted butter added	96	408	21.4	1.2	0	340	350	22	0.4	
fried in batter purchased cooked	199	834	19.6	10.3	7.5	100	370	80	0.5	
smoked poached in milk, butter added	101	426	21.6	1.6	0	1200	360	25	0.5	
Haddock steamed, unsalted	98	417	22.8	0.8	0	120	320	55	0.7	
Plaice fried in crumbs egg, unsalted	228	951	18.0	13.7	8.6	220	280	67	0.8	
steamed, flesh only, unsalted	93	392	18.9	1.9	0	120	280	38	0.6	
Herring grilled, flesh only, unsalted	199	828	20.4	13.0	0	170	370	33	1.0	

Salmon steamed flesh only, unsalted	197	823	20.1	13.0	0	110	370	29	0.8
Sardines canned in oil	217	906	23.7	13.6	0	650	430	550	2.9
Crab boiled in fresh water, meat only	127	534	20.1	5.2	0	370	270	29	1.3
Fish fingers frozen	178	749	12.6	7.5	16.1	320	240	43	0.7
fried	233	975	13.5	12.7	17.2	350	260	45	0.7

Vegetables

Asparagus boiled soft tips only, unsalted	18	75	3.4	Tr	1.1	2	240	26	0.9	1.5
Beans										
runner boiled, unsalted	19	83	1.9	0.2	2.7	1	150	22	0.7	3.4
broad boiled, unsalted	48	206	4.1	0.6	7.1	20	230	21	1.0	4.2
butter boiled, unsalted	95	405	7.1	0.3	17.1	16	400	19	1.7	5.1
baked canned in tomato sauce	64	270	5.1	0.5	10.3	480	300	45	1.4	7.3
Beetroot boiled, no skin, unsalted	44	189	1.8	Tr	9.9	64	350	30	0.4	2.5
Brussels sprouts boiled, unsalted	18	75	2.8	Tr	1.7	2	240	25	0.5	2.9
Cabbage										
spring boiled, unsalted	7	32	1.1	Tr	0.8	12	110	30	0.5	2.2
white raw	22	93	1.9	Tr	3.8	7	280	44	0.4	2.7
winter boiled, unsalted	15	66	1.7	Tr	2.3	4	160	38	0.4	2.8
Carrots										
old raw	23	98	0.7	Tr	5.4	95	220	48	0.6	2.9
boiled, unsalted	19	79	0.6	Tr	4.3	50	87	37	0.4	3.1
young canned	19	82	0.7	Tr	4.4	280	84	27	1.3	3.7
Cauliflower boiled, unsalted	9	40	1.6	Tr	0.8	4	180	18	0.4	1.8
Celery boiled, unsalted	5	21	0.6	Tr	0.7	67	130	52	0.4	2.2
Lentils split, boiled, unsalted	99	420	7.6	0.5	17.0	12	210	13	2.4	3.7
masur dahl, cooked	90	380	4.9	3.1	11.4	320	150	11	1.7	2.4

| Food | Energy value | | Protein | Fat | Carbohydrate | Sodium | Potassium | Calcium | Iron | Dietary fibre |
	kcal	kJ	g	g	g			mg		g
Lettuce raw	12	51	1.0	0.4	1.2	9	240	23	0.9	1.5
Marrow boiled, unsalted	7	29	0.4	Tr	1.4	1	84	14	0.2	0.6
Mushrooms raw	13	53	1.8	0.6	0	9	470	3	1.0	2.5
Onions boiled, unsalted	13	53	0.6	Tr	2.7	7	78	24	0.3	1.3
Parsnips boiled, unsalted	56	238	1.3	Tr	13.5	4	290	36	0.5	2.5
Peas										
frozen boiled, unsalted	41	175	5.4	0.4	4.3	2	130	31	1.4	12.0
canned processed	80	339	6.2	0.4	13.7	330	170	27	1.5	7.9
chick Bengal cooked, dahl	144	610	8.0	3.3	22.0	850	400	64	3.1	(6.0)
channa dahl	97	407	5.3	4.5	9.5	480	260	30	1.8	5.2
Peppers green raw	15	65	0.9	0.4	2.2	2	210	9	0.4	0.9
Potatoes										
old boiled, unsalted	80	343	1.4	0.1	19.7	3	330	4	0.3	1.0
roast, unsalted	157	662	2.8	4.8	27.3	9	750	10	0.7	—
chips, unsalted	253	1065	3.8	10.9	37.3	12	1020	14	0.9	—
instant powder	318	1356	9.1	0.8	73.2	1190	1550	89	2.4	16.5
made up	70	299	2.0	0.2	16.1	260	340	20	0.5	3.6
crisps	533	2224	6.3	35.9	49.3	550	1190	37	2.1	11.9
Swedes boiled, unsalted	18	76	0.9	Tr	3.8	14	100	42	0.3	2.8
Sweetcorn, canned kernels	76	325	2.9	(0.5)	16.1	310	200	3	0.6	5.7
Sweet potatoes boiled, unsalted	85	363	1.1	0.6	20.1	18	300	21	0.6	2.3
Tomatoes raw	14	60	0.9	Tr	2.8	3	290	13	0.4	1.5
fried, unsalted	69	288	1.0	5.9	3.3	3	340	15	0.5	3.0
Turnips boiled, unsalted	14	60	0.7	0.3	2.3	28	160	55	0.4	2.2
Yam boiled, unsalted	119	508	1.6	0.1	29.8	17	300	9	0.3	3.9

Fruit

Apples, eating (weighed with skin and core)	35	151	0.2	Tr	9.2	2	92	3	0.2	2.0
Avocado pears, flesh only	223	922	4.2	22.2	1.8	2	400	15	1.5	2.0
Bananas raw (weighed with skin)	47	202	0.7	0.2	11.4	1	210	4	0.2	2.0
Currants, black raw	28	121	0.9	Tr	6.6	3	370	60	1.3	8.7
Dates dried (weighed with stones)	213	909	1.7	Tr	54.9	4	650	58	1.4	7.5
Figs, dried raw	213	908	3.6	Tr	52.9	87	1010	280	4.2	18.5
Grapes, black (whole grapes weighed)	51	217	0.5	Tr	13.0	1	270	4	0.3	0.3
Grapefruit, raw (whole fruit weighed)	11	45	0.3	Tr	2.5	1	110	8	0.1	0.3
canned	60	257	0.5	Tr	15.5	10	79	17	0.7	0.4
Lemon juice, fresh	7	31	0.3	Tr	1.6	2	140	8	0.1	0
Melons, yellow, honeydew raw (weighed with skin)	13	56	0.4	Tr	3.1	12	140	9	0.2	0.6
Oranges (weighed with peel and pips)	26	113	0.6	Tr	6.4	2	150	31	0.3	1.5
juice, fresh	38	161	0.6	Tr	9.4	2	180	12	0.3	0
Pears, eating (weighed with skin and core)	29	125	0.2	Tr	7.6	1	94	6	0.1	1.7
canned fruit & syrup	77	327	0.4	Tr	20.0	1	90	5	0.3	1.7
Pineapple canned, fruit & syrup	77	328	0.3	Tr	20.2	1	94	13	0.4	0.9
Plums, Victoria dessert raw (weighed with stones)	36	153	0.5	Tr	9.0	2	180	10	0.3	2.0
Raspberries raw	25	105	0.9	Tr	5.6	3	220	41	1.2	7.4
Strawberries raw	26	109	0.6	Tr	6.2	2	160	22	0.7	2.2
Sultanas dried	250	1066	1.8	Tr	64.7	53	860	52	1.8	7.0

Food	Energy value kcal	kJ	Protein g	Fat g	Carbohydrate g	Sodium	Potassium	Calcium (mg)	Iron	Dietary fibre g
Nuts										
Almonds, weighed without shell	565	2336	16.9	53.5	4.3	6	860	250	4.2	14.3
Chestnuts, weighed without shell	170	720	2.0	2.7	36.6	11	500	46	0.9	6.8
Peanuts weighed without shell	570	2364	24.3	49.0	8.6	6	680	61	2.0	8.1
roasted and salted	570	2364	24.3	49.0	8.6	440	680	61	2.0	8.1
Peanut butter, smooth	623	2581	22.6	53.7	13.1	350	700	37	2.1	7.6
Walnuts, weighed without shell	525	2166	10.6	51.5	5.0	3	690	61	2.4	5.2
Sugars and preserves										
Sugar white	394	1680	Tr	0	105.0	Tr	2	2	Tr	0
Syrup golden	298	1269	0.3	0	79.0	270	240	26	1.5	0
Treacle black	257	1096	1.2	0	67.2	96	1470	500	9.2	0
Preserves										
Honey in jars	288	1229	0.4	Tr	76.4	11	51	5	0.4	0
Jam fruit with edible seeds	261	1114	0.6	0	69.0	16	110	24	1.5	1.1
Marzipan almond paste	443	1856	8.7	24.9	49.2	13	400	120	2.0	6.4
Mincemeat	235	1163	0.6	4.3	62.1	140	190	30	1.5	3.3
Confectionery										
Boiled sweets	327	1397	Tr	Tr	87.3	25	8	5	0.4	0
Chocolate milk	529	2214	8.4	30.3	59.4	120	420	220	1.6	—
plain	525	2197	4.7	29.2	64.8	11	300	38	2.4	—

Pastilles	253	1079	5.2	0	61.9	77	40	40	1.4	—
Toffees mixed	430	1810	2.1	17.2	71.1	320	210	95	1.5	—

Beverages

Coffee infusion, 5 minutes	2	8	0.2	Tr	0.3	Tr		2	Tr	
instant	100	424	14.6	0	11.0	41	66	160	4.4	
Horlicks malted milk	396	1679	13.8	7.5	72.9	350	4000	230	1.8	
Ovaltine	378	1606	9.8	3.8	81.2	150	750	36	2.6	
Tea, Indian, infusion 2–10 minutes	<1	2	0.1	Tr	Tr	Tr	850	Tr	Tr	
Coca-cola	39	168	Tr	0	10.5	8	17	4	Tr	
Lemonade bottled	21	90	Tr	0	5.6	7	1	5	Tr	
Lucozade	68	288	Tr	0	18.0	29	1	5	0.1	
Ribena undiluted	229	976	0.1	0	60.9	20	86	9	0.5	

Alcoholic beverages

	Alcohol g/100 ml									
Canned beer bitter	3.1	32	132	0.3	Tr	2.3	9	37	8	0.01
Lager bottled	3.2	29	120	0.2	Tr	1.5	4	34	4	Tr
Stout bottled	2.9	37	156	0.3	Tr	4.2	23	45	8	0.05
Cider dry	3.8	36	152	Tr	0	2.6	7	72	8	0.49
Red wine	9.5	68	284	0.2	0	0.3	10	130	7	0.90
Rosé medium	8.7	71	294	0.1	0	2.5	4	75	12	0.95
White wine, sweet, Sauternes	10.2	94	394	0.2	0	5.9	13	110	14	0.58
Port	15.9	157	655	0.1	0	12.0	4	97	4	0.40
Sherry medium	14.8	118	489	0.1	0	3.6	6	89	9	0.53
Curacao, Liqueur	29.3	311	1303	Tr	0	28.3	—	—	—	—
Spirits 70% proof	31.7	222	919	Tr	0	Tr	Tr	Tr	Tr	Tr

| Food | Energy value | | Protein | Fat | Carbo-hydrate | mg | | | | Dietary fibre |
	kcal	kJ	g	g	g	Sodium	Potassium	Calcium	Iron	g
Sauces and pickles										
Chutney tomato	154	658	1.1	0.1	39.7	130	310	30	1.1	1.9
Salad cream	311	1288	1.9	27.4	15.1	840	80	34	0.8	—
Tomato ketchup	98	420	2.1	Tr	24.0	1120	590	25	1.2	—
Soups										
Bone and vegetable broth	60	251	3.7	4.6	1.1	74	64	17	0.3	—
Chicken, cream of canned, ready to serve	58	242	1.7	3.8	4.5	460	41	27	0.4	—
Minestrone dried, as served	23	99	0.8	0.7	3.7	430	62	9	0.2	0.5
Oxtail canned, ready to serve	44	185	2.4	1.7	5.1	440	93	40	1.0	—
dried, as served	27	116	1.4	0.8	3.9	400	54	11	0.3	0.3
Tomato, cream of canned, ready to serve	55	230	0.8	3.3	5.9	460	190	17	0.4	—
dried, as served	31	130	0.6	0.5	6.3	390	89	14	0.2	0.3

Index

317